The Survivor's Handbook
Eating Right for Cancer Survival

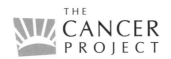

THE
CANCER
PROJECT

5100 Wisconsin Avenue, N.W., Suite 400
Washington, D.C. 20016
www.CancerProject.org

ISBN 0-9761919-0-3

COVER PHOTO © STOCKBYTE
COVER SUBJECT IS A MODEL USED FOR
ILLUSTRATIVE PURPOSES ONLY

Printed in USA

Updated
February 2005

The Cancer Project proudly displays the Humane Charity Seal of Approval.

A Note to the Reader

The *Survivor's Handbook: Eating Right for Cancer Survival* was written by Neal D. Barnard, M.D., with the help of Jennifer K. Reilly, R.D. It was developed to accompany The Cancer Project's "Nutrition and Cooking Classes for Cancer Survivors" series. However, it is sufficiently detailed to be used on its own and will give you important insights into food's role in cancer prevention and cancer survival.

Our goal is to provide you with information about foods and health. However, neither this book nor any other can take the place of individualized medical care or advice. All cancer treatments, including diet changes, must take into account your needs as an individual. In addition, if you are overweight, have any health problem, or are on medication, you should consult with your doctor before making any changes in your diet or exercise routines, and you should follow your doctor's recommendations, which will be based on your personal needs.

There are many situations in which a diet change can alter your need for medications. For example, individuals with diabetes, high blood pressure, or high cholesterol levels often need less medication when they improve their diets. You should be sure to work with your physician to adjust your regimen as needed.

The science of nutrition grows gradually as time goes on, so we encourage you to consult other sources of information, including the references listed in this volume.

With any dietary change, it is important to ensure complete nutrition. Be sure to include a source of vitamin B_{12} in your routine, which could include any common multivitamin, fortified soymilk or cereals, or a vitamin B_{12} supplement of five micrograms or more per day.

We wish you the very best of health.

Contents

INTRODUCTION

How Foods Fight Cancer

For many years, researchers have been investigating how food choices can help prevent cancer and, when cancer has been diagnosed, how these choices can improve survival. While their work is by no means finished, what is already known is nothing short of dramatic. Certain diet patterns seem to have a major effect, helping people diagnosed with cancer to live longer, healthier lives. Other diet choices are risky propositions, increasing the toll cancer takes.

Our goal is to translate scientific findings into simple, practical steps you can use in your own kitchen, at the grocery store, at restaurants—anywhere you're thinking about what to eat. We'll divide this information into eight sections and include key scientific information, meal-planning tips, and suggested steps you can take at home. We will also list recipes that illustrate the key points in each section. Some recipes embody more than one nutritional advantage, so we'll list especially good ones in more than one section. All the recipes (and more) are included in the back of this book.

Before we begin, one note of caution: As we explore the role of food in cancer, some people might feel a bit uneasy. If foods can affect cancer risk, they ask, does that mean I am somehow to blame for my illness? Did the foods I ate as a child cause this problem? Is our culture causing these problems?

It is, of course, only natural that concerns like these will cross our minds. However, let us encourage you to set blame aside. The fact is, some people do their very best to follow healthy lifestyles and still develop cancer. And you may have known people who smoke, drink heavily, and eat with absolute abandon and yet manage to live to a ripe old age. Unfortunately, it is easy to get cancer, and we cannot predict with certainty who will be affected by it and who will not. So let's focus not on blame but on what foods can do for you. As Jack Nicklaus used to say, you can spend all day trying to figure out why you hit your ball into the woods—or you can just go in and get it out.

Research into food's role in cancer survival grew from studies looking at the causes of the illness. As researchers compared the diets of people who developed cancer and those of people who remained healthy, finding many factors that do indeed influence cancer risk, they also had an opportunity to look forward, seeing how various eating patterns affect survival.

It turns out that many foods that help prevent cancer in the first place also seem to help us beat the disease when it has struck. Among the most important themes to emerge from research has been the fact that foods influence hormones that fuel cancer growth. For example, diets that are very low in fat tend to reduce the amount of estrogens (female sex hormones) circulating in the bloodstream. That turns out to be a good thing, because taming estrogens seems to reduce the likelihood that cancer cells will multiply or spread. It is not just low-fat foods that help in this way. Fiber-rich foods reduce estrogens, too, and also reduce the amount of testosterone in the blood, which is of key importance in prostate cancer.

Many parts of the diet can help us stay healthy or regain health when we're dealing with illness. Vegetables, fruits, beans, soy products, and many other foods have been under study for some time. While we do not have all the answers, we have more than enough information to get started with healthier ways of eating.

As we begin, let us encourage you not to simply dabble with diet changes. If you or a loved one have been diagnosed with a major illness, it's time to take full advantage of what diet can do for you. Much as we might like to pretend that small diet changes help, the fact is that trimming a little fat here and adding a piece of fruit there does very little. That has been proven true in studies using diet to control cholesterol, diabetes, hypertension, osteoporosis, weight problems, and many other conditions. So we will not sell you short with half-baked dietary suggestions, and we will encourage you to jump in and take full advantage of what these foods can offer.

Chances are, you will love where you're headed. An exploration of healthy eating can not only bring you better health; it can also lead to new and interesting tastes, exotic restaurants, and some of the most remarkable aisles in the grocery store.

Yes, you'll have some challenges along the way. A new recipe might turn out stunningly or it could also be a dud. Don't worry. That's what experimenting is all about. But as you get to know what works for you, you'll discover a new world of healthy, powerful foods and delicious tastes, not to mention an entirely new way of thinking about food and health.

Fueling Up on Low-Fat Foods

Many teams of researchers have studied the health of various populations around the world, hoping to tease out the causes of cancer and ways to prevent it. In one study after another, they have found that people following plant-based diets tend to have strikingly low cancer rates. In rural Asia and Africa, for example, traditional diets are based on rice or other grains, starchy vegetables, fruits, and beans, and people eating these diets generally avoid the disease. When it does strike, they also seem to have better survival.

When these populations trade their traditional diets for a menu based on Western foods—either because they have migrated or because fast-food restaurants and other Western food purveyors have come to them—their cancer rates promptly change. In Japan, dramatic diet changes began after World War II. Traditional rice dishes were gradually replaced with hamburgers. Dairy products, which had been almost unknown in Japan, became popular. Carbohydrate intake fell, and fat consumption soared. Soon, cancer rates began to rise, as did the toll of obesity, heart problems, and other diseases.

Although many factors may be at work here, let us focus first on one key biological fact: Fatty foods boost the hormones that promote cancer. Specifically, diets rich in meat, dairy products, fried foods, and even vegetable oils cause a woman's body to make more estrogen.* In turn, that extra estrogen increases cancer risk in the breast and other organs that are sensitive to female sex hormones.

To see why this matters, think for a moment about estrogen's role in the body. In simple terms, estrogen makes things grow. As an adolescent girl develops a mature figure, she experiences estrogen's ability to stimulate the growth of breast tissue. The hormone also thickens the lining of the uterus every month as a woman's body prepares for the possibility of pregnancy.

Estrogen not only makes normal tissues grow. It can also make cancer cells grow. When researchers add a bit of estrogen to breast cancer cells in a test tube, they multiply rapidly. And, in fact, one of the main goals of breast cancer treatment is to reduce estrogen's effects (using drugs, such as tamoxifen, that block estrogen's activity).**

> Fatty foods boost the hormones—estrogen and testosterone—that promote cancer.

---

* The term *estrogen* actually refers to a group of hormones, including estradiol, estrone, and others. For simplicity, they will be referred to here as "estrogen."

** Although researchers have long known that estrogens encourage the *growth* of cancer cells once they form, evidence also suggests that they can also spark the very first step in cancer development: the transformation of healthy cells into cancer cells. Specifically, enzymes in the body alter estrogens to produce other molecules that can damage DNA, leading to cancer.[1]

Here is where diet comes in. Foods influence estrogen's effect, too—to a striking degree. When a woman begins a low-fat diet, the amount of estrogen in her blood drops almost immediately. In a matter of weeks, the amount in her bloodstream drops by 15 to 50 percent, depending on how low in fat her diet is.[2,3] She will still have more than enough estrogen for fertility, but she will nonetheless have less estrogen than before. From the cancer prevention standpoint, that's a good thing. It means there will be less stimulus for cancer cell growth.

A 2003 study published in the *Journal of the National Cancer Institute* found that when girls aged eight to ten reduced the amount of fat in their diet—even very slightly—their estrogen levels were held at a lower and safer level during the next several years. When the girls increased intake of vegetables, fruits, grains, and beans and reduced intake of animal-derived foods, the amount of estradiol (a principal estrogen) in their blood dropped by 30 percent, compared to a group of girls who did not change their diets.[4]

The same phenomenon occurs in men. Men have estrogen in their blood, too—although much less than women have—and cancer researchers have long suspected that both estrogen and testosterone (the "male hormone") play roles in prostate cancer risk. But as men cut the fat from their diets, the amounts of both estrogen and testosterone tend to fall. Don't worry—this change does not make a man any less masculine. But it may well reduce the hormonal stimulus for prostate cancer growth.

Because of these and related findings, many researchers have suggested that steering clear of meat, dairy products, fried foods, and other fatty fare may reduce cancer risk. However, it is important to understand that in order to reduce cancer risk or effectively change its course, diet changes have to be significant. Studies have shown that modest diet changes do little or nothing. Indeed, large studies of American women have shown that moderate variations in their fat intake make no difference in their breast cancer risk. The best evidence suggests that, to be effective, diet changes have to be fairly profound.

Nonetheless, research bears out a major effect of diet, not only on cancer prevention, but also on cancer survival. Breast cancer patients who follow lower-fat diets do tend to live substantially longer. Researchers at the State University of New York in Buffalo tracked the diets of 953 women who had been diagnosed with breast cancer. They then followed them to see who did well and who did not. The results were striking. The risk of dying at any point in time increased by 40 percent for every 1,000 grams of fat the women consumed per month.[5] To see what this means in practical terms: If you were to add up all the fat in a typical American diet over the course of a month and compare it to the amount of fat in a low-fat, pure vegetarian diet, the two would differ by approximate 1,500 grams of fat each month. If the study's findings hold, that would correspond to a 60 percent increased risk of dying at any point in time for patients following a typical American diet.

Several other studies have found much the same thing: Women with breast cancer who eat fattier foods—meats, dairy products, and fried foods—have greater rates of cancer recurrence and succumb more fre-

> The risk of dying at any point in time increased by 40 percent for every 1,000 grams of fat the women consumed per month.

quently than do those whose diets are based on the lower-fat choices—vegetables, fruits, whole grains, and beans.[6] Frightening as this sort of finding may be, it shows us a path toward reducing the need for further treatment and improves the odds of living a life free of the tolls cancer can take.

Similar findings have emerged regarding prostate cancer. Men on healthier diets—that is, diets rich in vegetables, fruits, and other low-fat foods from plant sources—are less likely to develop cancer in the first place and, if cancer does strike, more likely to survive it.[7-9]

Chicken Is Not a Vegetable

Many people try to trim fat from their diets by switching from beef to chicken. Unfortunately, chicken has nearly as much fat as beef. As you'll see in the table below, the leanest beef is 28 percent fat (as a percentage of calories). The leanest chicken—skinless breast meat, prepared without added fat—is not much better, at about 23 percent. Fish vary, with some lower than chicken and some higher, but the truly low-fat foods are in a class by themselves: Beans, vegetables, fruits, and whole grains are virtually all very low in fat and, as we'll see in later sections, high in vitamins, minerals, and healthy fiber.

Fat in Foods (PERCENTAGE OF CALORIES)

Atlantic salmon	40
Beef, round bottom, lean	29
Chicken, white meat, skinless	23
Tuna, white	21
Broccoli	8
Rice, brown	8
Apple	6
Beans, navy	3
Lentils	3
Orange	2

If you or your loved ones are trying to eliminate fat from your diet, switching from beef to chicken does not bring you very far. On the other hand, building your menu from whole grains, beans, vegetables, and fruits is a powerful way to trim the fat.

We'll conclude this section with the results from a surprising experiment conducted at the University of California at Los Angeles. Researchers drew blood samples from a group of men who had been following a low-fat diet and exercising regularly for several years. They also drew blood samples from overweight men who were not following any diet or exercise program. They then added portions of each man's blood serum to test tubes

Building your menu from whole grains, beans, vegetables, and fruits is a powerful way to trim the fat.

containing standardized prostate cancer cells. It turned out that serum from men on the low-fat diet and exercise program *slowed cancer cell growth* by 49 percent, compared to serum from the other men. The changes in diet and exercise had caused the amount of testosterone, estrogen, and other components in the blood to change so dramatically that the effect on cancer cells was obvious right in the test tube.[10]

The effect occurs quickly. The research team found cancer-inhibiting power within as little as eleven days after beginning a low-fat diet and exercise regimen.[11]

Cutting down on fat is an important first step in preventing cancer and in surviving it if it has been diagnosed. So how do we go about it? The easiest way is to build your meals from foods that are naturally low in fat and to use cooking methods that don't require you to add fats or oils. In the next session, we'll see how to begin.

Meal Planning: The New Four Food Groups

The easiest and perhaps most useful guide to basic nutrition is called the *New Four Food Groups*, introduced by the Physicians Committee for Responsible Medicine in 1991. Let's briefly review its guidelines; then, we will see how the guidelines turn into actual meals.

The New Four Food Groups are vegetables, legumes, fruits, and whole grains. The idea is to build your diet by choosing a variety from each of these groups. Here are suggestions for the number of servings from each group:

- Vegetables: 3 or more servings per day
- Legumes (beans, peas, and lentils): 2 or more servings per day
- Whole grains: 5 or more servings per day
- Fruits: 3 or more servings per day
- Add any common multiple vitamin to ensure adequate intake of vitamin B_{12}

The suggested serving numbers are just suggestions to get you started. Feel free to vary your proportions as you like. For example, one way of using the New Four Food Groups follows a traditional Asian pattern, favoring grains, such as rice or noodles, with smaller amounts of vegetables and bean dishes, and reserving fruit for dessert. However, it is just as acceptable to emphasize more vegetables and fewer grain products. Some people who gravitate toward raw foods will increase fruits. You can get complete and healthful nutrition using essentially any pattern that uses each of the four groups.

For optimal nutrition, you will want to avoid meat (red meat, poultry, and fish), dairy products, eggs, added oils, and high-fat foods (potato chips, olives, nuts and nut butters, seeds, and avocados). Steer clear of fried foods and any oily or fatty toppings, such as margarine or typical salad dressings (non-fat dressings are fine). Avoiding fatty foods helps your taste buds to reduce their preference for greasy tastes. When you select breads, cereals, or other grain products, favor those that retain their normal fiber (e.g., brown rice rather than white rice).

So how does all this translate into actual meals? The foods you'll now focus on are not really so different from what you already eat. Breakfast might be a big bowl of old-fashioned oatmeal with cinnamon and raisins (but skip the milk). If you like, add some cantaloupe or whole-grain toast. Lunch might be a bowl of split pea soup or perhaps a plate of baked beans with crackers. Dinner could be minestrone followed by angel hair pasta with marinara sauce—or perhaps an autumn stew of vegetables, beans, and hearty grains.

Recommended Recipes

Hummus (page 83)
Easy Bean Salad (page 96)
Easy Stir-Fry (page 117)
Breakfast Shakes (page 139)

To Do This Week:
Check Your Diet with a 3-Day Dietary Record

You can get a good idea of the healthfulness of your overall diet with a three-day dietary record. This is the same diet-tracking tool researchers use in clinical studies. It not only lets you see exactly what you're eating now, it also helps you see how to improve your diet over time. If, for example, you're getting a little too much fat or too little fiber, you'll spot it right away and can fix the problem.

To do your record, you simply take a sheet of paper, and note down *everything* you eat or drink (except water) for three days, including two weekdays and one weekend day (most of us eat a bit differently on weekends, compared to weekdays).

Using the Diet Record form on page 15 (photocopy it as many times as you need to), jot down each food, condiment, or beverage on a separate line. For example, if you had a salad made of lettuce, tomatoes, chickpeas, and dressing, use four lines, one for each ingredient. Or if you had a peanut butter and jelly sandwich, along with a cola, use four lines so you can separate out each part of the meal—bread, peanut butter, jelly, and the drink.

Write down everything you eat, including snacks and condiments. The only item to omit is water. Record the amount of each food as accurately as you can. You can either weigh each item using a food scale (available in stores that sell kitchenware) or measure or estimate its volume (e.g., one cup of orange juice, or perhaps a small, medium, or large apple).

Record your foods as you go so you don't forget. If it is more convenient, you can keep notes in a small notebook and transfer them to the Diet Record form later. Be thorough.

If you like, you can get a detailed nutrient analysis of your diet. Just be sure to fill in quantities carefully and use a food scale. A dietitian can analyze the record for you, or you can simply log onto a nutrient analysis Web site, such as the University of Illinois' Food Science and Human Nutrition Department's site, *www.nat.uiuc.edu/mainnat.html*, or *www. dietsite.com.* Please note that while the nutrient analyses on these sites are accurate, their nutrition guidelines are not necessarily optimal. Many commonly used guidelines allow too much fat and cholesterol. Here is a better set of goals: For an adult consuming 2,000 calories per day, a good fat intake goal is about 25–35 grams each day. This works out to about 10–15 percent of calories. Cholesterol intake should be zero. Your protein intake should be roughly 50 grams per day. Resist the temptation to push protein intake too high.

Section 1 References

1. Miller K. Estrogen and DNA damage: the silent source of breast cancer? J Natl Cancer Inst 2003;95:100-2.

2. Prentice R, Thompson D, Clifford C, Gorbach S, Goldin B, Byar D. Dietary fat reduction and plasma estradiol concentration in healthy postmenopausal women. The Women's Health Trial Study Group. J Natl Cancer Inst 1990;82:129-34.

3. Heber D, Ashley JM, Leaf DA, Barnard RJ. Reduction of serum estradiol in postmenopausal women given free access to low-fat high-carbohydrate diet. Nutrition 1991;7:137-9.

4. Dorgan JF, Hunsberger SA, McMahon RP, et al. Diet and sex hormones in girls: findings from a randomized controlled clinical trial. J Natl Cancer Inst 2003;95:132-41.

5. Gregorio DI, Emrich LJ, Graham S, Marshall JR, Nemoto T. Dietary fat consumption and survival among women with breast cancer. J Natl Cancer Inst 1985 Jul;75(1):37-41.

6. Chlebowski RT. Dietary fat reduction in postmenopausal women with primary breast cancer: Phase III Women's Intervention Nutrition Study (WINS). Paper presented at: American Society of Clinical Oncology Annual Meeting; May 16, 2005; Torrance, CA.

7. Fradet Y, Meyer F, Bairati I, Shadmani R. Dietary fat and prostate cancer progression and survival. Eur Urol 1999;388:91.

8. Carter JP, Saxe GP, Newbold V, Peres CE, Campeau RJ, Bernal-Green L. Hypothesis: Dietary management may improve survival from nutritionally linked cancers based on analysis of representative cases. J Am Coll Nutr 1993;12:209-26.

9. Saxe GA, Hebert JR, Carmody JF, et al. Can diet in conjunction with stress reduction affect the rate of increase in prostate specific antigen after biochemical recurrence of prostate cancer? J Urol 2001;266:2202-7.

10. Tymchuk CN, Barnard RJ, Ngo TH, Aronson WJ. Role of testosterone, estradiol, and insulin in diet- and exercise-induced reductions in serum-stimulated prostate cancer cell growth in vitro. Nutr Cancer 2002;42:112-6.

11. Tymchuk CN, Barnard RJ, Heber D, Aronson WJ. Evidence of an inhibitory effect of diet and exercise on prostate cancer cell growth. J Urol 2001;166:1185-9.

Diet Record

Make as many copies of this page as you need. Record only one ingredient per line.

Date: _____

Time of day	Food	Amount	Cooking method

SECTION 2

Favoring Fiber

Earlier, we saw how low-fat foods can tame the hormones that fuel the growth of common forms of cancer. As you'll recall, cutting the fat from your diet reduces the amount of estrogen and testosterone in the bloodstream. But in addition to reducing how quickly your body *makes* hormones, you can also augment your body's ability to rid itself of them— that is, to eliminate waste hormones. It all depends on fiber. And fiber has other important benefits, too, as we'll see in this section.

Fiber is another word for plant roughage—the part of beans, grains, vegetables, and fruits that resists digestion. Fiber helps keep you regular by moving the intestinal contents along. But it has another equally important role. It helps us rid ourselves of all manner of chemicals—including hormones—that our bodies are anxious to dispose of.

This "waste disposal" system starts in your liver, which continuously filters your blood. As blood passes through the liver's network of tiny capillaries, liver cells remove toxins, cholesterol, medications, waste hormones, and whatever else your body figures it is better off without. These undesirables are then sent from the liver into a small tube, called the bile duct, which leads to your intestinal tract. There, fiber soaks up these chemicals and carries them out with the wastes.

Now, there is plenty of fiber in vegetables, fruits, beans, and whole grains. So if these are a big part of your diet, your "waste disposal" system works pretty well. The liver pulls hormones out of the bloodstream, they slide down the bile duct, fiber picks them up, and out they go.

But what happens if your lunch consisted of a chicken breast and a cup of yogurt? These products don't come from plants—and that means they have no fiber at all. Not a speck. So when your liver sends hormones or other chemicals into the intestinal tract, there is nothing for them to attach to. They end up being *reabsorbed back into your bloodstream*, and the whole process starts over again. This endless cycle—hormones passing from the bloodstream, through the liver, into the intestinal tract, and, unfortunately, back into the bloodstream—is called *enterohepatic circulation*. It keeps hormones circulating for longer than they should. Fiber stops this cycle by carrying hormones out once and for all.

> The liver pulls hormones out of the bloodstream, they slide down the bile duct, fiber picks them up, and out they go.

Fiber versus Colon Cancer

Fiber has another function you should know about. It may reduce your risk of colon cancer. Fiber moves intestinal contents along, so that whatever carcinogens (that is, cancer-causing chemicals) may be lurking in your waste products are escorted out of the body more quickly.

Carcinogens don't just come from factory waste and air pollution. They are sometimes present in foods. For example, when chicken, fish, or red meat is cooked at a high temperature, cancer-causing chemicals called *heterocyclic amines* tend to form as the protein molecules and other parts of muscle tissue are deformed by the intense heat. Needless to say, that is another good reason to avoid these products. However, the bile your body produces to digest fats can also encourage the production of carcinogens. A high-fiber diet helps move these compounds out of your body.

Aim for 40 Grams per Day

So where do you find the fiber you need? Animal products don't have any. That goes for red meat, poultry, fish, eggs, and dairy products, which is why people who center their diets on these foods often struggle with constipation. On the other hand, plant products in their natural state have quite a lot of fiber, which is why vegetarians rarely have any need for laxatives. The first key to building a high-fiber diet is to eat plenty of vegetables, fruits, beans, and whole grains and to avoid animal products.

But a meaty diet is not the only wrong turn you can make. Let's say that for breakfast you had a choice between old-fashioned oatmeal with whole-grain toast on the one hand, and a bagel and jam on the other. The first breakfast is loaded with fiber. But a bagel has very little. It is made from white flour—that is, wheat flour whose fiber has been removed in the refining process. Refining makes it soft and white but leaves it almost devoid of fiber.

If you choose whole-grain bread instead of white bread, you'll get much more fiber. The same is true for brown rice, which retains the grain's tan-colored outer layer, as opposed to white rice, which has lost this high-fiber layer in the refining process.

Generally speaking, the most fiber-rich foods are beans and vegetables, followed by fruits and whole grains. Yes, breakfast cereals and other grain products advertise their high fiber content. But you'll find surprisingly large amounts of it in simple bean and vegetable dishes.

Fiber comes in two forms:

Soluble fiber is the kind that dissolves in water, in the way that oatmeal, for example, gets creamy as it cooked. There is also plenty of soluble fiber in beans, barley, and several other foods. Soluble fiber is especially known for its ability to control cholesterol levels.

Insoluble fiber, which is found in wheat, rice, and many other grains, is visibly different. Rice or wheat grains just don't get "gooey" the way oatmeal does. Insoluble fiber is especially helpful for keeping the intestinal contents moving along and fighting constipation.

From the standpoint of cancer prevention, you'll want to get both kinds. If your diet is rich in beans, vegetables, fruits, and whole grains, you'll get plenty of healthy fiber. An average American gets only 10–15 grams of fiber

When chicken, fish, or red meat is cooked at a high temperature, cancer-causing chemicals called *heterocyclic amines* tend to form.

per day. Health authorities would like to see that number rise significantly. A sensible and easily reached goal is 40 grams per day. Having said that, you may wish to reach this goal gradually, rather than in one jump. It may take a few weeks for your digestive tract to get used to the change.

Whole grains, such as brown rice and old-fashioned oatmeal, are pretty easy to digest. You'll find that cruciferous vegetables, such as broccoli, cabbage, and cauliflower, are easier to digest if they are cooked until soft. If beans cause gas for you, start with smaller quantities, be sure they are well-cooked, and try different varieties.

Quick Fiber Check

The Quick Fiber Check is a handy little tool. Using its simple scoring concept, which takes only a minute or two to learn, you'll be able to estimate the fiber content of virtually everything in the grocery store and calculate your own fiber intake.

To check your meals, write down everything you eat or drink for one full day on the form that follows. Next to each food, jot in its fiber score, using the following guide:

Beans: For each half-cup serving of beans or lentils or any food that includes about this amount of beans or lentils as an ingredient, mark 7. One cup of soymilk or one-half cup of tofu rates 3.

Vegetables: For each one-cup serving of vegetables, mark 4. An exception is lettuce, for which one cup scores 2. A potato with skin scores 4; without the skin, it scores 2.

Fruit: For each medium piece of fruit (e.g., apple, orange, banana, one cup of apple sauce, a banana smoothie), mark 3. For one cup of juice, mark 1.

Grains: For each piece of white bread, bagel, or equivalent, score 1. Whole grain breads score 2. One cup of cooked pasta scores 2. One cup of rice scores 1 for white and 3 for brown. One cup of cooked oatmeal scores 4. Score 3 for typical ready-to-eat cereals, 1 for highly processed and colored cereals, and 8 for bran, or check package information.

Meat, poultry, or fish: Score 0. Animal products do not contain fiber.

Eggs or dairy products: Score 0.

Sodas, water: Score 0.

Quick Fiber Check

Food (one food or ingredient per line):	Fiber Score
_____	_____
_____	_____
_____	_____
_____	_____
_____	_____
_____	_____
_____	_____
_____	_____
_____	_____
_____	_____
_____	_____
_____	_____
_____	_____
_____	_____
_____	_____
_____	_____
_____	_____
_____	_____
Total	_____

Interpreting Your Quick Fiber Check Score

Less than 20: You need more fiber in your diet. As it is, your appetite will be hard to control, and you may have occasional constipation. Boosting fiber will help tame your appetite and can cut your risk of many health problems.

20–39: You are doing better than most people in Western countries, but as you bring more fiber into your diet, you will find that it makes foods more satisfying and cuts your calorie intake a bit.

40 or more: Congratulations. You have plenty of healthy fiber in your diet. It tames your appetite and helps keep you healthy. Fiber also reduces your risk of cancer, heart disease, diabetes, and digestive problems.

High-Fiber Cooking

Beans Are the Fiber Champions

Beans are loaded with fiber. If you are using canned beans, you can reduce their sodium content by choosing reduced-sodium brands or draining the liquid and rinsing the beans before serving them. If you use dried beans, you'll avoid added sodium, although cooking is usually more time-consuming.

Taming the Wild Bean: Easing Digestion

If beans give you a bit of indigestion or gas, here are some tips that will solve this problem:

1. After soaking dried beans, drain them, and then cook them in fresh water. It may also help to add a pinch of baking soda to the soaking water.

2. Make sure the beans are thoroughly cooked. Adding a strip of kombu, a sea vegetable, to the beans during cooking can also be helpful.

3. Drain and gently rinse canned beans. This also decreases the amount of salt in some brands.

4. Start with modest servings. Also, some people notice that smaller beans are easier to digest, so try black beans, black-eyed peas, and lentils first, and then work your way up to pinto and fava beans.

5. Commercial enzyme products help in the digestion of complex carbohydrates. The most common and widely available product is called Beano. A few drops added to cooked beans right before eating them won't change the taste and may help in digestion.

Cooking Yield of Dried Beans

Variety	Water/ Bean Ratio	Cooking Time After Soaking	Cooked Quantity of 1 Cup Dried Beans After Soaking
Black (turtle) beans	3:1	1½ hours	3 cups
Black-eyed peas	3:1	30 minutes	2½ cups
Chickpeas (garbanzos)	4:1	1½ hours	3 cups
Kidney beans	3:1	1 to 1½ hours	2¾ cups
Lentils, brown	2:1	30 minutes	3 cups
Lentils, red	2:1	15 to 20 minutes	3 cups
Lima beans	3:1	1 hour	3 cups
Mung beans	3:1	45 minutes	3 cups
Navy (pea) beans	3:1	45 to 60 minutes	2¾ cups
Pinto beans	3:1	45 minutes	3¼ cups
Soybeans	4:1	2 hours	2¾ cups

Source: *Moosewood Restaurant Low-Fat Favorites*, Clarkson Potter publishers, 1996

Recommended Recipes

Basic Brown Rice (page 101)
Quick Bean Burritos (page 121)
Tomato Corn Salsa (page 85)
Guacamole Plus (page 83)
Calabacitas (page 103)

To Do This Week

Drop by any large grocery store, and take a look at the beans. You'll notice they are found in three different aisles. First, you'll find bags of dried beans in a surprising range of varieties. Then, in the canned vegetables section, you'll find baked beans, limas, and other types. And in the "ethnic" or "international" aisle, you'll find Italian varieties (e.g., chickpeas, cannellini beans), Mexican refried beans, and perhaps other types. Select at least one new bean variety or product, and give it a try this week. If you're not too big on beans, start with small servings to avoid gassiness.

While you're there, pick up a package of whole-grain rice—that is, brown rice. Brown rice retains the natural grain fiber that is missing from white rice. Try the simple cooking method in the recipe section (Basic Brown Rice, page 101).

Discovering Dairy Alternatives

Most North Americans and Europeans grow up with the idea that milk is a healthful beverage, and the dairy industry has certainly done its best to promote that idea. However, researchers seeking to understand why people following Western diets tend to have high cancer rates have begun to point a finger of blame not only at meat and other fatty foods, but also at dairy products.

In 1998, Harvard researchers reported findings in a large group of health professionals. Those who typically had more than two servings of milk per day had a 60 percent increased risk of prostate cancer, compared to those who generally avoided milk.[1] Two years later, another Harvard study on a separate large group of men showed much the same thing—milk-drinkers had significantly more prostate cancer.[2] Many other studies have had similar findings, and researchers have also examined the role of dairy products—positive or negative—in other forms of cancer.

What is all this about? Why should dairy products influence cancer risk? Is the problem due to hormones or other chemicals in milk, or is it due to the basic nutrient makeup of milk—its fat or protein, perhaps? What does this mean for people who have been diagnosed with cancer already? And if milk does have health risks, what do we replace it with?

Milk Promotes Growth of Infants—and Cancer Cells

To understand why dairy products might play a role in cancer, it helps to remember its biological purpose, so to speak. Milk is produced by mothers to support the rapid growth of their newborns. It contains plenty of protein, fat, and sugar (lactose), as well as dozens of hormones and other natural chemical substances that direct infants' growth and development. Milk differs from species to species—cow's milk is quite different in its nutrient profile from human milk—but all mammals' milk is designed to encourage rapid growth.

After the age of weaning, of course, all mammals stop drinking their mothers' milk. A few thousand years ago, however, humans began to consume milk taken from cows and a few other mammals. Until relatively recently (in the historical sense), this curious practice was limited to northern Europe and a few other places.

When humans drink cow's milk, it causes some worrisome biological changes in the body, one of which is a rise in the amount of *insulin-like growth factor I* (IGF-I) in the bloodstream.[3,4] IGF-I is a powerful stimulus for cancer cell growth. When breast cancer cells are mixed with IGF-I in a test tube, for example, they grow rapidly.

Researchers have known for many years that men and women with higher levels of IGF-I in their blood are at significantly higher risk for prostate and premenopausal breast cancer, respectively, compared to those with lower levels.[5,6] So one way that milk may influence cancer risk is by increasing the amount of IGF-I in the blood. Individuals who have been diagnosed with cancer may be quite right to be concerned that milk drinking boosts IGF-I levels in their bloodstreams, given that IGF-I, in turn, can encourage cancer cell growth.

Milk causes other chemical changes in the body as well, some of which relate to specific types of cancer. Generally speaking, these mechanisms relate not only to the likelihood that cancer will strike, but also to how rapidly it will grow and spread once it has occurred.

Prostate Cancer

As we've seen, large studies have shown that milk-drinking men have a higher risk of prostate cancer. However, milk's ability to boost IGF-I is not the only mechanism by which this occurs. Milk fat, like the other fats you read about in Section 1, may also increase the body's production of testosterone, which is linked to prostate cancer risk.

In addition, milk appears to interfere with the activation of vitamin D in the body. Vitamin D is actually a hormone that helps your body absorb calcium from the digestive tract. It also protects the prostate against cancer. It is normally produced by sunlight's action on the skin, and it can also come from the diet. However, these forms of the vitamin are inactive precursors. In order to function as full-fledged vitamin D, they must pass first to the liver and then to the kidneys for slight changes to their molecular structure.

And this is where dairy products become a problem. As the load of calcium in dairy products floods into the bloodstream, it apparently signals the body that, since there is plenty of calcium in the system already, the body does not need to activate vitamin D to try to absorb any more. That is, the body reduces its vitamin D activation so that it does not absorb *too much* calcium, since calcium overdoses can be toxic.

The result of all this is that high-calcium foods can cause a substantial drop in the amount of activated vitamin D in the blood. And, since vitamin D is essential for maintaining a healthy prostate, less vitamin D in the blood may mean that the risk of prostate cancer climbs. Indeed, researchers have found that less vitamin D in the blood is indeed associated with higher cancer risk. Of course, milk often contains some added vitamin D, but it is in the inactive precursor form, and dairy consumption actually suppresses vitamin D activation in the body.[1]

At least 16 research reports in diverse populations, including the

Milk-drinkers have more IGF-I in their bloodstreams. IGF-I is a powerful stimulus for cancer cell growth.

People with cancer may be quite right to be concerned that milk drinking boosts IGF-I levels in their bloodstreams, given that IGF-I, in turn, can encourage cancer cell growth.

Harvard studies mentioned above, have linked milk drinking to prostate cancer.

Other Cancers

Researchers at Harvard University and elsewhere have studied the links between milk consumption and ovarian cancer, with mixed results. The hypotheses under scrutiny have related not only to milk's fat content, but also to its sugar, *lactose.*

Lactose is actually made of two smaller sugar molecules, called *galactose* and *glucose*. When these two sugars are split apart—either by the bacteria used to produce yogurt or by digestive enzymes in your intestinal tract—galactose and glucose enter the blood. And galactose may be the problem. In large concentrations, galactose may be toxic to the ovaries, encouraging infertility and possibly cancer. A recent analysis of studies examining a relationship between dairy product consumption (skim, low-fat, and whole milk, yogurt, cheese, and total lactose [dairy sugar]) and ovarian cancer risk found that for every 10 grams of lactose consumed (the amount in one glass of milk), ovarian cancer risk increased by 13 percent among the prospective cohort studies.[6]

With regard to breast cancer, women with higher levels of IGF-I in their blood have a greater risk of premenopausal breast cancer. The Harvard Nurses' Health Study found that women with higher IGF-I levels had more than double the risk, compared to women with lower IGF-I levels.[7] Other researchers have made similar findings.[8] As we've seen, milk-drinking raises IGF-I levels.

Other studies seeking to nail down the links between dairy consumption and breast cancer risk have yielded mixed results, with some finding higher risk of breast cancer among milk-drinkers and others finding no such association.

Foods that are high in calcium appear to reduce colon cancer risk. However, people seeking ways to use calcium-rich foods to reduce colon cancer risk would do well to get their calcium from green leafy vegetables and beans rather than from dairy products. Prostate and breast cancer are much more common than colon cancer. Using dairy products to try to reduce colon cancer risk may increase the risk of other, much more common cancers.

Healthier Beverages

There is no shortage of better beverages. Soymilk, rice milk, almond milk, and oat milk come in a wide variety of flavors and work very well on cereal or for drinking. They are available in calcium-fortified and regular versions, and many have vitamin fortification. Because many varieties require no refrigeration until opened, groceries sometimes stock them on the regular shelves rather than in the refrigerated section.

The Healthiest Calcium Sources

Green leafy vegetables and legumes (beans, peas, and lentils) contain calcium, and, unlike milk, are rich in fiber and other nutrients that protect against cancer. You'll also find plenty of calcium in supplements and, as we've seen, in fortified soymilk. Calcium-fortified juices are now widely available. However, it is important to remember that increased calcium intake may be one of the reasons why milk is linked to prostate cancer (because high calcium intakes interfere with vitamin D activation). If that is true, you should be equally cautious about *any* product that is extremely high in calcium (i.e., fortified foods or supplements). In that light, green leafy vegetables and beans are your best calcium sources. They have adequate calcium, but not excessive amounts.

However, don't depend on calcium—from any source—to protect you from osteoporosis. While the dairy industry has pushed drinking milk as a means of preventing the bone-thinning condition, studies show that the strategy is largely useless.

Researchers at Pennsylvania State University found that, in girls in their peak bone-building years—ages 12 to 18—getting extra calcium made no difference at all in bone growth.[9] Exercise worked very well to foster bone growth, but extra calcium did not. Similarly, in the Nurses' Health Study, a group of nearly 78,000 women followed for 12 years showed that dairy calcium didn't help bone strength at all. Women who got the most calcium from dairy sources actually had nearly double the hip fracture rates, compared to those who got little or no dairy calcium.[10]

So how do you protect your bones? Here are the most important factors to remember:

- Exercise, of course, is the first key. Your bones need a reason to live, so to speak—and exercise strengthens them noticeably.

- Vitamin D—from sunlight or vitamin supplements—helps keep bones strong.

- Fruits and vegetables provide vitamin C to build collagen, which forms the basic network of tissue within your bones.

Perhaps most important of all, you should understand that osteoporosis is not a condition of inadequate calcium intake, for the most part. Rather, *it is a condition of overly rapid calcium loss.* Three factors, in particular, accelerate calcium losses, and controlling them gives you important power against osteoporosis:

- Sodium (salt) accelerates the passage of calcium through the kidneys into the urine. To reduce sodium intake, avoid adding salt in cooking or at the table, and be careful about canned foods and snack products made with added sodium.

- Animal protein is high in *sulfur-containing amino acids*, which tend to leach calcium from the bones and send it through the kidneys into the urine.

- Smokers have rapid calcium losses.

Calcium in Plant Foods

Food	Serving size	Calcium content (mg)	Percentage of calcium absorbed	Estimated absorbable calcium/ serving (mg)
Almonds, dry roasted	1 ounce	80	21	17
Beans, navy	1 cup	121–128	17	21–22
Beans, white	1 cup	161	17	27
Broccoli, boiled	1 cup	178	53	94
Brussel sprouts, boiled	1 cup	56	64	36
Chinese cabbage (bok choy), boiled	1 cup	158	54	85
Cabbage, green, boiled	1 cup	50	65	33
Cauliflower, boiled	1 cup	34	69	23
Figs, dried	5 medium	135	n/a	n/a
Kale, boiled	1 cup	94	59	55
Mustard greens, boiled	1 cup	104	58	60
Orange juice, calcium-fortified	8 fluid ounces	300	38	114
Rice milk, calcium-fortified	8 fluid ounces	300	24	72
Sesame seeds, unhulled	1 ounce	381	21	58
Soymilk, calcium-fortified	1 cup	300	24	72
Spinach, boiled	1 cup	244	5.1	12
Tofu, calcium-set, firm	½ cup	258	31	80
Total® Cereal	¾ cup	1000	30	300
Turnip greens, boiled	1 cup	198	52	103

Sources:

Weaver CM, Proulx WR, Heaney R. Choices for achieving adequate dietary calcium with a vegetarian diet. Am J Clin Nutr. 1999;70(suppl):543S-548S.

Weaver CM, Plawecki KL. Dietary calcium: adequacy of a vegetarian diet. Am J Clin Nutr. 1994;59(suppl):1238S-1241S.

Keller JL, Lanou AJ, Barnard ND. The consumer cost of calcium from food and supplements. J Am Diet Assoc. 2002;102:1669-71.

Meal Planning

- Include calcium-rich greens (kale, collards, mustard greens, turnip greens, bok choy, Swiss chard, etc.) and beans in your routine. Add greens and/or beans to stir-fries, sauces, salads, and casseroles.
- Have calcium-rich snacks, such as figs, raisins, almonds, and dates.

- Replace cow's milk with rice milk, almond milk, or oat milk in meals and recipes.
- Sprinkle nutritional yeast on pasta and other main dishes for a healthy cheesy alternative to regular cheese.
- Try fresh fruit sorbets and non-dairy frozen desserts instead of ice cream or frozen yogurt.
- Enjoy oatmeal and other calcium-rich breakfast cereals with fresh fruit and rice milk for breakfast.

Recommended Recipes

Creamy Spinach Dip (page 82)
Braised Collards or Kale (page 102)
Penne with Fresh Spinach, Tomatoes, and Olives (page 121), topped with nutritional yeast
Store-bought lemon or raspberry sorbet for dessert

To Do This Week

Did you ever switch from whole milk to skim or nonfat milk? How did the new version taste at first? For many people, fat-reduced milks taste watery and a bit "off" at first. But after two or three weeks, what happened? The new milk tasted perfectly fine, didn't it? And if you ever went back to whole milk, what was it like then? Chances are, it seemed too thick and fatty—almost like paint.

It takes only a couple of weeks for your tastebuds to accommodate to new tastes. So if you try rice milk or another non-dairy beverage, it will probably not taste quite right at first. But within a couple of weeks, it will taste perfectly fine.

This week, take a trip to the health food store (or a large, well-stocked grocery store). If you normally drink milk or add it to cereal, pick up a few different brands of rice milk and give them a try. Notice they come in regular, vanilla, chocolate, and perhaps other flavors, as well as low-fat varieties and other products enriched with vitamins and calcium.

If you are a fan of yogurt, ice cream, sour cream, or cheese, don't worry. Health food stores stock non-dairy substitutes for them, too. Some are more flavorful than others, so try a few different varieties and see which ones appeal to you.

Section 3 References

1. Giovannucci E, Rimm EB, Wolk A, et al. Calcium and fructose intake in relation to risk of prostate cancer. Cancer Res 1998;58:442-7.

2. Chan JM, Stampfer MJ, Ma J, Gann PH, Gaziano JM, Giovannucci E. Dairy products, calcium, and prostate cancer risk in the Physicians' Health Study. Am J Clin Nutr 2001;74:549-54.

3. Cadogan J, Eastell R, Jones N, Barker ME. Milk intake and bone mineral acquisition in adolescent girls: randomised, controlled intervention trial. BMJ;1997;315:1255-60.

4. Heaney RP, McCarron DA, Dawson-Hughes B, et al. Dietary changes favorably affect bone remodeling in older adults. J Am Dietetic Asso 1999;99:1228-33.

5. Cohen P. Serum insulin-like growth factor-I levels and prostate cancer risk—interpreting the evidence. J Natl Cancer Inst 1998;90:876-9.

6. Larsson SC, Orsini N, Wolk A. Milk, milk products, and lactose intake and ovarian cancer risk: A meta-analysis of epidemiological studies. Int J Cancer: published online 28-July-05.

7. Hankinson SE, Willett WC, Colditz GA, et al. Circulating concentrations of insulin-like growth factor I and risk of breast cancer. Lancet 1998;351:1393-6.

8. Peyrat JP, Bonneterre J, Hecquet B, et al. Plasma insulin-like growth factor-1 (IGF-1) concentrations in human breast cancer. Eur J Cancer 1993;29A:492-7.

9. Lloyd T, Chinchilli VM, Johnson-Rollings N, Kieselhorst K, Eggli DF, Marcus R. Adult female hip bone density reflects teenage sports-exercise patterns but not teenage calcium intake. Pediatrics 2000;106:40-4.

10. Feskanich D, Willett WC, Stampfer MJ, Colditz GA. Milk, dietary calcium, and bone fractures in women: a 12-year prospective study. Am J Publ Health 1997;87:992-7.

SECTION 4

Replacing Meat

Whenancer researchers started to search for links between diet and cancer, one of the most noticeable findings was that people who avoided meat were much less likely to develop the disease. Large studies in England and Germany showed that vegetarians were about 40 percent less likely to develop cancer, compared to meat-eaters.[1–3] In the United States, researchers studied Seventh-day Adventists. This religious group is remarkable because, although nearly all members avoid tobacco and alcohol and follow generally healthful lifestyles, about half of the Adventist population is vegetarian, while the others consume fairly modest amounts of meat. This fact allowed scientists to separate the effects of eating meat from other factors. Overall, these studies showed significant reductions in cancer risk among those who avoided meat.[4]

At Harvard University, researchers zeroed in on red meat, finding that individuals eating beef, pork, or lamb daily have approximately three times the colon cancer risk, compared to people who generally avoid these products.[5–6]

Why Is Meat Linked to Cancer?

Why should meat contribute to cancer risk? For starters, its fat content is virtually always much higher than that of plant products. As we saw in Section One, fatty foods boost the hormones that are linked to common forms of cancer. Even skinless chicken breast harbors a surprising amount of fat, and virtually all meats are totally out of the league of truly low-fat foods—whole grains, beans, vegetables, and fruits.

And, since meat is not a plant product, it never has any fiber at all. The more you fill up on meat, the less room you have for fiber-rich foods. It is also devoid of vitamin C and low in other protective nutrients found in plants.

But meat has other problems. As meats are cooked, cancer-causing chemicals called *heterocyclic amines* tend to form within the meat tissue, as we saw in Section 2. The longer and hotter it is cooked, the more these compounds form. Chicken is by no means exempt from this problem. In some studies, grilled chicken has turned out to have high concentrations of these cancer-causing substances.[7]

Large research studies have shown that vegetarians are about 40 percent less likely to develop cancer, compared to meat-eaters.

Healthier Protein Sources

Some people think of meat as their main source of protein. But it is easy to get plenty of protein without the fat, cholesterol, and other undesirables in meat.

Beans, vegetables, and whole grains, in particular, have more than enough protein. The American Dietetic Association holds that a diet that includes a variety of these healthy plant foods provides all the protein you need.[8] In years past, some people thought that vegetarians had to eat foods in certain combinations—grains with beans, for example—in order to get adequate protein. However, it turns out that no special combining is necessary. A diet including a variety of beans, vegetables, and whole grains will easily give you more than enough protein, even without intentional combining of foods.

> The American Dietetic Association holds that a diet that includes a variety of healthy plant foods provides all the protein you need.

Meal Planning

So how do we replace meat? In many recipes, the legume group comes to your rescue. Beans and lentils, for example, add heartiness to soups, stews, chili, and other recipes. When making burritos, leave out the ground beef and use vegetarian refried beans. Despite their name, low-fat "refried" beans are not really fried. They are actually just mashed pinto beans. You'll find them in the Mexican food section of your local grocery store. They're filling and loaded with fiber and protein, and you'll never miss the meat.

Portabello mushrooms also make great meat alternatives. They have a meaty texture and savory flavor, especially after being marinated in low-fat dressing and then grilled or heated in a frying pan. Use portabello mushrooms as "burgers" at your next barbecue or to fill the meat layer in your lasagna.

Seitan is a fascinating product derived from wheat protein. It has been used to simulate virtually every kind of cold cut or meaty dish imaginable. It has a hearty texture and makes a healthy meat substitute. Wheat protein is also the main ingredient in a number of meat analogs, including spicy veggie pepperoni and sausages.

Soy products have been turned into endless varieties of hot dogs, burgers, and other simulated meats. Many of these products taste so much like the real thing that they will help you break a meat habit. Properly chosen, they will also greatly reduce the fat content of your diet. Some researchers have suggested that soy has special cancer-fighting properties, although investigations in this area are not yet sufficient to support this possibility. For now, soy's proven virtue is its ability to pry people away from meat; its overall effect on cancer risk is not yet established.

Recommended Recipes

Asian Fusion Salad (page 94)
Pan-Grilled Portabello Mushrooms (page 105)
Buckwheat Pasta with Seitan (page 115)
Tempeh Broccoli Sauté (page 126)

To Do This Week

1. Check out meat substitutes at a health food store and try one or more of them. Try a sampling of veggie burgers, hot dogs, and deli slices or, if you prefer, the many varieties of beans and lentils.

2. Turn three of your favorite recipes into meatless meals using beans, seitan, mushrooms, tofu, tempeh, or other meat substitutes.

Section 4 References

1. Thorogood M, Mann J, Appleby P, McPherson K. Risk of death from cancer and ischaemic heart disease in meat and non-meat eaters. Br Med J 1994;308:1667-70.

2. Chang-Claude J, Frentzel-Beyme R, Eilber U. Mortality patterns of German vegetarians after 11 years of follow-up. Epidemiology 1992;3:395-401.

3. Chang-Claude J, Frentzel-Beyme R. Dietary and lifestyle determinants of mortality among German vegetarians. Int J Epidemiol 1993;22:228-36.

4. Barnard ND, Nicholson A, Howard JL. The medical costs attributable to meat consumption. Prev Med 1995;24:646-55.

5. Willett WC, Stampfer MJ, Colditz GA, Rosner BA, Speizer FE. Relation of meat, fat, and fiber intake to the risk of colon cancer in a prospective study among women. N Engl J Med 1990;323:1664-72.

6. Giovannucci E, Rimm EB, Stampfer MJ, Colditz GA, Ascherio A, Willett WC. Intake of fat, meat, and fiber in relation to risk of colon cancer in men. Cancer Res 1994;54:2390-7.

7. Sinha R, Rothman N, Brown ED, et al. High concentrations of the carcinogen 2-amino-1-methyl-6-phenylimidazo-[4,5] pyridine [PhIP] occur in chicken but are dependent on the cooking method. Cancer Res 1995;55:4516-19.

8. American Dietetic Association. Position of the American Dietetic Association: vegetarian diets. J Am Diet Asso 1997;97:1317-21.

Planning Healthy Meals

You now have the basic knowledge and cooking skills you need to begin to make some major changes in your eating habits. There is much more to learn, of course, but now's the time to put what you know to work. In this section, you'll have a chance to experience what it is like to be on as perfect a diet as possible. We will use a unique method to learn new tastes and break away from bad habits. Along the way, we will also look at what to do when you do not have complete control over the menu, for example, at restaurants or fast-food outlets.

The Three-Week Break

The best and easiest way to try a new way of eating is to take what you might call a "three-week break." That is, select a three-week period and, during this time, build your meals only from the best possible foods while setting aside unhealthy foods completely. At the end of three weeks, see how you feel. If you like how things are going—if you've lost a few pounds and are feeling healthier and more energetic—you can stick with it. If, however, this just doesn't feel right to you, you are free to go back to your old way of eating. Your diet experiment lasts only three weeks, and remembering that fact will help you to give it your all.

Do not do it halfway. Now is the time to jump in and really see what healthy eating feels like. If, instead, you were to just have an occasional healthy, vegetarian meal now and then while continuing to have meaty, cheesy dishes at other times, you would keep reminding your taste buds of the very foods that cause health problems and would never lose your taste for these foods. Let yourself have a clean break and really try healthy foods on for size.

In Section 3, we talked about the common experience of switching from whole milk to skim or nonfat brands to illustrate how quickly we adjust to lighter tastes. Well, now is your chance to lighten up your entire menu. At first, your taste buds might miss fatty foods, but that will soon pass as they come to embrace healthier choices.

Your taste buds have a memory of about three weeks. So whether you are looking to cut the fat from your diet, reduce salt, break a sugar habit, or get to know truly healthy foods, using a three-week break—and really doing it all the way—gives you the momentum you need.

> Your taste buds have a memory of about three weeks. So using a three-week break—and really doing it all the way—gives you the momentum you need.

Use the New Four Food Groups

During your three-week break, we'll use the nutrition-planning guide called the New Four Food Groups, which we got to know in Section 1. Let's briefly review these guidelines. Choose foods from these four groups:

- Vegetables: 3 or more servings per day

- Legumes (beans, peas, and lentils): 2 or more servings per day

- Whole grains: 5 or more servings per day

- Fruits: 3 or more servings per day

- Add any common multiple vitamin to ensure adequate intake of vitamin B_{12}

The suggested serving numbers are just suggestions to get you started. Feel free to vary your proportions as you like. One handy way to do this is to let grains fill up about half your plate, vegetables one quarter, and a bean dish the remaining quarter. Let fruit be a dessert or snack. However, if you would like to pile the vegetables high and reduce the grains, that's perfectly fine. Feel free to enjoy more than one type of vegetable at your meal—say, an orange vegetable, such as yams, with a green vegetable, such as broccoli.

Making It Work

A note of caution: Merely *resolving* to eat right doesn't work very well. It's too easy to slip off track. To make sure it really does work for you, you need to do a few things:

First, *plan* what you will eat. Use the form on the next page or any handy sheet of paper (yes, really do it), marking down "breakfasts," "lunches," and "dinners." Under each heading, list foods that meet the New Four Food Groups guidelines and that work for you.

Second, *go out and buy* these foods so they're in your kitchen when you need them.

Third, and most important, *throw away everything else*. If you're threatened by a serious illness, unhealthy foods are not your friends. Get rid of them.

Okay, let's get started. If you're testing out new recipes, expect that some will turn out better than you would have expected and some might have the opposite result. Don't worry. That's what experimenting is all about.

Meal Planning

Breakfasts

_____

_____

_____

_____

_____

Lunches

_____

_____

_____

_____

_____

Dinners

_____

_____

_____

_____

_____

Restaurants and Fast Food

More and more of our meals are served at restaurants, and much of what's on the menu is far from healthy. But that doesn't mean you have to forego dining out. If you're a little choosy about which restaurants you patronize and about what you order when you arrive, you'll find plenty of great options.

For starters, it helps to think international. Restaurants that feature the cuisines of other lands often have a broad range of healthful menu items. For example, at an Italian restaurant, you'll find minestrone, pasta and bean soup, pasta with marinara or pesto sauce, and green vegetables sautéed with garlic. Chinese and Thai restaurants have plenty of savory soups, along with "vegetable" dishes, which are actually main dishes made from tofu, broccoli, spinach, green beans, and other ingredients. You'll also find a great many rice and noodle dishes. Ask them to use their more traditional cooking methods, without the added oil that may Westerners have come to expect. Japanese restaurants serve miso soup, salads, appetizers, and vegetable sushi, all of which are usually very low in fat and delicately prepared.

Mexican restaurants serve bean burritos, which, if prepared without lard and not smothered in cheese, are usually low in fat and free of cholesterol. Indian restaurants always feature many delicious vegetarian choices, from appetizers to desserts. Ask the waiter to skip the dairy products and to be careful about the overzealous use of oil.

At American restaurants and steak houses, you'll find salad bars and vegetarian plates. More and more fast food and family-style restaurants now feature veggie burgers, salad bars, and baked potato bars.

Recommended Recipes

Salad of Color (page 99)
Quickie Quesadillas (page 121)
Breakfast Scramble (page 136)
Berry Applesauce (page 129)

To Do This Week

The 3-3-3 Way to Revamp Your Diet

If you're going to stick to healthy foods for three weeks—or for the rest of your life—you don't have to be a gourmet chef. If you think about it, most of us choose our dinner on any given night from only about eight or nine different favorite meals that make up our culinary repertoires. So, when you're revamping your menu, all you need are eight or nine *healthy* meals that you like. Once you've found them, you've got everything you need.

Try this: Jot down on a piece of paper the names of three meals you already like that contain no animal products and are reasonably low in fat. For example, you might choose pasta with a marinara sauce, a bean and rice burrito filled with grilled vegetables, a garden salad with kidney beans and low-fat Italian dressing, a portabello mushroom sandwich with roasted red peppers, or veggie chili with crackers.

Next, write down three more meals you like that could be easily modified to eliminate animal products and added fat. Examples might include a vegetable stew instead of the beefy variety, a stir-fry with vegetables instead of chicken, a chili made with beans and chunky vegetables instead of meat, or a hamburger using a veggie burger patty instead of the usual patty.

Finally, write down three meals that are new to you that you'd like to try. Take a look at the recipes in the back of this book for ideas and pick out three that appeal to you.

Now, if you have done this exercise thoughtfully, you've found nine meals that are likely to work for you, and you have just solved your problem. There are many other great foods to try, of course, but you are off to a tremendous start.

SECTION 6

Antioxidants and Phytochemicals

As you push your grocery cart down the aisle, you'll want to keep a lookout for foods that have special cancer-fighting properties. In this chapter, we'll focus on foods rich in protective compounds called *antioxidants* and *phytochemicals*. If these names sound a bit technical, don't worry; you'll soon know what they are and where to find them.

These cancer fighters are mainly found in vegetables and fruits. While we'll look in some detail at which vegetables and fruits are high in which protective compounds, the key message is *to be generous with a variety of vegetables and fruits* as you plan your menu. Studies have amply demonstrated the ability of diets rich in vegetables and fruits to reduce the likelihood that cancer will develop in the first place. And although fewer studies have investigated their effect on survival after diagnosis, some have suggested that cancer survivors who consume more vegetables and fruits do indeed live longer. As you'll see, researchers have begun to tease out reasons why this is so.[1,2]

Antioxidants

To understand antioxidants, let's start with how oxygen works in the body. Every minute of every day, we breathe in oxygen and breathe out carbon dioxide. Although oxygen is used for a variety of vitally important functions in the body, it happens to be a very unstable molecule. In the course of the normal chemical reactions that occur in the bloodstream or inside our cells, oxygen can easily be damaged, which is to say it can lose some of its electrons or perhaps gain some. And while electrons normally orbit a molecule's nucleus in as calm and orderly a fashion as the moon circles Earth, oxygen's electrons can slip into off-kilter orbits.

The point is that we have millions of oxygen molecules in our bodies, and they easily become unstable. When that happens, they become like piranhas, ready to take a bite out of the cells that make up your skin, blood vessels, internal organs, or any other part of your body. These piranhas—these unstable and dangerous oxygen molecules—are called *free radicals*. They can even attack your *chromosomes*, the strands of DNA that lie deep within your cells and hold all the genes that make you who you are. When oxygen free radicals damage chromosomes, cells can lose their ability to control their basic functions. They can begin to multiply out of control—and that is the beginning of cancer. Biologists believe that much of the aging process and many cancers are caused by free radical damage.

Plants can be damaged by oxygen free radicals, too. So nature has given them the ability to produce natural compounds that act like shields to defend against these wild oxygen molecules. You can see why these natural compounds are called "antioxidants"—they protect the plant from oxygen free radicals. And when you eat plants, their antioxidants enter your bloodstream and act to protect you, too. When all goes well, the free radicals—the unstable oxygen molecules—attack the antioxidants and leave your cells and chromosomes alone in the same way that a bullet might dent the hardened surface of an armored car but spare the occupants inside.

Beta-Carotene

One of the best-known antioxidants is *beta-carotene*, the yellow-orange pigment found in carrots, yams, and cantaloupes. Beta-carotene has long been looked on kindly by nutritionists because it provides vitamin A, which is important for good vision, among other functions. Beta-carotene is actually two molecules of vitamin A joined together.

However, beta-carotene does more than simply provide vitamin A. It enters the cell membrane that surrounds each of the cells that make up your body and then waits there to fend off free radicals that might approach.

You'll find beta-carotene not only in orange-colored vegetables, but also in dark green vegetables. You can't see it, because their chlorophyll hides beta-carotene in the same way that chlorophyll in tree leaves hides the plants' underlying orange, red, and brown colors until the green color fades in autumn.

While you can buy beta-carotene supplements, it is much better to get beta-carotene from foods. In fact, studies testing beta-carotene's cancer-fighting power in smokers (a group selected because they are at particular risk for cancer) showed that those whose diets were high in beta-carotene had a measure of protection, but those who got beta-carotene from supplements were actually *more likely to develop cancer* than were other smokers. The reason is not entirely clear, but it may be that, since supplements deliver high doses of only one antioxidant, they interfere with the absorption of others. Also, vegetables and fruits that are rich in beta-carotene are also loaded with hundreds of other antioxidants, vitamins, minerals, and other protective compounds.

The moral of the story is that there is plenty of beta-carotene in vegetables and fruits, and they are the best sources. On the following page are some top foods for beta-carotene:

Beta-carotene enters the cell membrane that surrounds each of your cells and protects the cell from free radicals.

Beta-Carotene (mg)

Cantaloupe (1 cup)	3
Carrot (1 large)	16
Kale (1 cup)	4
Mango (1 cup)	4
Pumpkin (1 cup)	32
Yam (1 cup)	26

Lycopene

You may not have heard much about *lycopene*, but you have certainly seen plenty of it. Just as beta-carotene is nature's yellow-orange pigment, lycopene is a bright red pigment, providing the color for tomatoes, watermelon, and pink grapefruit.

Lycopene is in the *carotenoid* family, meaning that it is beta-carotene's chemical cousin, and it is actually a much more powerful antioxidant. A study at Harvard University showed that men who had just two servings of tomato sauce per week had 23 percent less prostate cancer risk, compared to those who rarely had tomato products.[3] Men consuming ten or more servings of tomato products each week had a 35 percent reduction in risk, and that was true *even if their tomatoes came in the form of pizza sauce, spaghetti sauce, or ketchup*. In fact, the cooking process releases lycopene from the plant's cells, increasing your ability to absorb it.

Not all red foods contain lycopene, however, as nature has a couple of other similar pigments in its paint box. The red color in strawberries, for example, does not come from lycopene, but from a group of pigments called *anthocyanins*, which are powerful antioxidants in their own right. (Other anthocyanins provide the color for cherries, plums, red cabbage, and blueberries.)

Here are the top foods for lycopene:

> Men who had ten or more servings of tomato products each week had 35 percent less prostate cancer risk.

Lycopene (mg)*

Pink grapefruit (1)	10
Tomato (1 medium, raw)	4
Tomato juice (1 cup)	25
Tomato ketchup (1 Tbsp)	3
Tomato-based spaghetti sauce (1 cup)	56
Watermelon (1 slice, 368 g)	15

*Source: Heinz Institute of Nutritional Sciences, *www.lycopene.org*.

Vitamin E and Selenium

Vitamin E and the mineral *selenium* are also part of your antioxidant arsenal. Like beta-carotene and lycopene, they protect each cell's outer membrane from free radical attacks. Vitamin E is found in legumes (beans), whole grains, and plants rich in natural oils (e.g., nuts, seeds).

However, while a little bit of vitamin E is good—in fact, it is an essential part of your body's protection against free radicals—it is not at all certain that boosting vitamin E intake to high levels is a good idea. Some of the richest vitamin E sources, such as vegetable oils and nuts, also give you an unwanted load of fat. This may be the reason why one study found that, among women with breast cancer, those with the highest levels of vitamin E in their bloodstreams were actually *more likely* to succumb to the disease than those with more moderate levels—it may simply be a sign that they were getting too much fat in their diets.[4] So while more research is needed to sort out what is the right amount of vitamin E, it is prudent to choose foods that are moderate in the vitamin, rather than extremely high or low. These foods are listed in the chart below.

The amount of selenium in plants varies depending on the amount present in the soil where they grow. But, given modern food distribution patterns, your rice is likely to come from one place, your beans from another, and so on. So your selenium intake is likely to be reasonably generous if you include grains and legumes in your daily routine.

Good Vitamin E and Selenium Sources
(portions are 1 cup raw, unless specified)

	Vitamin E (mg)	Selenium (mcg)
Barley (cooked)	3	36
Brown rice (cooked)	1	14
Broccoli	2	3
Brussels sprouts (cooked)	1	2
Garbanzo beans (cooked)	2	6
Garlic	0	19
Pumpkin (cooked)	3	1
Pinto beans (cooked)	2	12
Sunflower seeds (1 Tbsp)	5	5

Vitamin C

Vitamin C is a powerful and well-known antioxidant. But unlike the other antioxidants we've looked at so far, which defend cell membranes, vitamin C patrols the watery areas of the body—the bloodstream or the cell's interior.

What are the best foods for vitamin C? Well, citrus fruits are famous for it, but you'll find surprisingly large amounts in many vegetables. Here are some good sources:

Vitamin C (mg) (portions are 1 cup raw, unless specified)

Bell pepper, red	175
Broccoli	82
Brussels sprouts, cooked	97
Cantaloupe	68
Guava	303
Orange (1 medium)	59
Orange juice	124
Strawberries	82

Phytochemicals

While antioxidants have the job of protecting you from the free radicals, plants have many other protective substances, too. Biologists call them *phytochemicals*. "Phyto" comes from the Greek word "phyton," which means "plant," so phytochemicals are simply natural chemicals found in plants.

Although researchers first turned their attention to these chemicals because of their apparent ability to prevent cancer, the possibility that these natural compounds can also enhance survival after cancer has been diagnosed is also now under study. Two groups are especially good to get to know: *cruciferous* vegetables and the *allium* family of vegetables.

Cruciferous vegetables, such as broccoli, cabbage, and collard greens, get their name from the cross-shaped flowers that adorn them in the garden (but which are long gone by the time they reach the grocery store). People who eat generous amounts of these vegetables have remarkably low cancer rates, and researchers have dedicated a great deal of effort to isolating the compounds that are responsible for their anti-cancer effects.

Broccoli, for example, contains *sulforaphane*, a compound that augments the liver's ability to rid the body of toxic chemicals. Other phytochemicals in broccoli and other cruciferous vegetables have demonstrated the ability to arrest the growth of cancer cells.[2,5]

Cruciferous Vegetables

Arugula	Cabbage	Kohlrabi	Turnips
Beet greens	Cauliflower	Mustard greens	Turnip greens
Bok choy	Collard greens	Radishes	Watercress
Broccoli	Horseradish	Rutabaga	
Brussels sprouts	Kale	Swiss chard	

Cruciferous vegetables also affect the hormones that influence the progression of hormone-dependent cancers, such as breast cancer. In particular, these vegetables actually change the way estrogens are broken down and eliminated. Normally, estradiol—a potent estrogen in a woman's bloodstream—is converted to *16α-hydroxyestrone*, a hormone that encourages the growth of cancer cells. However, the cruciferous extract *indole-3-carbinol* causes the body to convert more estrogen to a different estrogen called *2-hydroxyestrone*, which has anticancer actions.[6]

Researchers are starting to test out the effects of cruciferous vegetable extracts on patients. In one study, the extract indole-3-carbinol was given to women with abnormal cervical cells (the type of cells gynecologists check for on Pap smears). After 12 weeks, the abnormal cells had disappeared in half the treated patients, while patients given a placebo preparation showed no improvement.[6]

Because some vegetables, such as broccoli, are difficult to digest in their raw state, you may be wondering if cooking knocks out their protective effects. Studies show that, while cooking does indeed reduce the amount of phytochemicals in vegetables, it does not eliminate them.[2]

The *allium* group of vegetables includes garlic, onions, and hundreds of their botanical relatives. Yes, chefs value their flavors, but researchers are increasingly intrigued by the possibility that they may speed the body's elimination of carcinogens and perhaps even block the start of cancer or inhibit the growth of cancer cells.

Garlic, in particular, has been subjected to a great deal of scientific study. When garlic cloves are cut or crushed, they produce a compound called *allicin*, which is responsible for both their scent and their biological activity. Several studies have shown that people who regularly include allium vegetables in their diets have less risk of cancer, particularly cancers of the stomach and colon.[7] In test-tube experiments, extracts from these plants have been shown to help the body eliminate carcinogens and slow the growth of cancer cells.[8] Researchers estimate the amount of garlic necessary for anti-cancer effects at three to five cloves daily.[9] Cooking temperatures eliminate garlic's beneficial effects on cells unless the garlic is allowed to stand for about 10 minutes between being crushed and the cooking process.[10]

Allium Vegetables

Chives	Onions
Garlic	Scallions
Leeks	Shallots

It should be noted that tests of garlic's ability to block cancer promotion have been carried out in cells, not in intact humans, so it remains to be established whether garlic can actually affect the course of cancer after diagnosis.

Antioxidants in Foods

Serving size = one cup raw unless otherwise specified.	Vitamin C mg*	Beta-carotene mcg**	Vitamin E mg	Selenium mcg
Daily target (minimum)	Women 75 mg Men 90 mg	Women 800 mcg Men 1000 mcg	15 mg	55 mcg
Vegetables				
Broccoli	82	807	1.5	3
Brussels sprouts, cooked	97	669	1.3	2
Cabbage	29	69	1.5	1
Carrot, large (4 oz), 1	11	15,503	0.7	1
Carrot juice	20	12,559	1	1
Cauliflower	46	12	0.1	1
Garlic (1 clove)	0.9	0	0	0.4
Kale	80	3,577	0.5	1
Leeks, cooked	4	31	0.7	1
Mushrooms	2	0	0.3	8
White onions, cooked	11	0	0.8	1
Potato, medium, baked, 1	16	0	0.1	1
Pumpkin, cooked	10	31,908	2.6	1
Red bell pepper	175	2,840	0.7	0.3
Spinach	8	1,196	0.8	0.3
Acorn squash, cooked	26	627	1.6	2
Sweet potato, cooked	49	26,184	0.6	1
Tomato, medium, 1 🍅	23	446	1.1	0.5
Orange yam, baked	49	26,184	0.6	1
Fruits				
Apple, medium, 1	8	28	0.9	0.4
Apricots, 3	10	1,635	0.9	0.4
Banana, medium	11	57	0.4	1.3
Blueberries	19	87	2.7	1
Cantaloupe (1/8 melon)	29	1,325	0.2	0.3
Cantaloupe, cubes	68	3,072	0.5	0.6
Grapefruit sections 🍅	79	160	0.6	3
Grapes	4	54	0.3	0.2
Guava	303	750	1.8	1
Kiwi fruit, 2	114	164	1.7	0.6
Mango	46	3,851	1.8	1
Orange, medium, 1	59	52	0.4	1
Orange juice	124	92	0.5	0.2
Papaya	87	70	1.6	0.8
Peach, 1	6	260	1	0.4
Raspberries	31	48	0.6	0.7
Strawberries	82	23	0.4	1
Watermelon 🍅	27	634	0.4	0.3

Antioxidants in Food (continued)

Serving size = one cup raw unless otherwise specified.	Vitamin C mg*	Beta-carotene mcg**	Vitamin E mg	Selenium mcg
Daily target (minimum)	Women 75 mg Men 90 mg	Women 800 mcg Men 1000 mcg	15 mg	55 mcg
Grains and Grain Products				
Barley, cooked	0	0	3	36
Brown rice, cooked	0	0	1.1	14
Millet, cooked	0	0	1.3	2
Oatmeal, cooked	0	0	0.2	19
Whole-wheat bread, 1 slice	0	0	0.3	10
Wheat germ, 2 Tbsp	0	0	2.6	11.4
Beans and Legumes				
Black beans, cooked	0	10	1	2
Black-eyed peas, cooked	1	20	0.5	4
Garbanzo beans, cooked	2	28	2	6
Kidney beans, cooked	2	3	0.4	2
Lentils, cooked	3	11	1.2	6
Pinto beans, cooked	4	2	1.6	12
Soybeans, cooked	3	10	3.4	13
Split peas, cooked	1	11	1.6	1
Tofu, firm	1	0	0.1	44
White beans, cooked	0	0	2	2
Nuts, Seeds, and Oils				
Almonds, ½ oz, 2 Tbsp, 12 nuts	0	0	3.8	1
Brazil nuts, ½ oz, 2 Tbsp, 3 nuts	0	0	1	420
Cashews, ½ oz, 2 Tbsp	0	0	1	2
Peanuts, ½ oz, 2 Tbsp, 17 nuts	0	0	1.1	1
Walnuts, ½ oz, 2 Tbsp, 7 halves	3	0	0.4	0.6
Flaxseed, 1 Tbsp	1	0	0.1	6
Sunflower seeds, 1 Tbsp	0	3	5	5
Olive oil, 1 tsp	0	0	0.6	0

*mg=milligram, 1/1,000 of a gram

**mcg= microgram, 1/1,000,000 of a gram

🍅 = rich in lycopene

Meal Planning

Here are some simple tips that will help you build generous amounts of antioxidants and phytochemicals into your diet:

- Include plenty of vegetables and fruits in your routine, emphasizing the colorful varieties.
- Keep a bag of baby carrots (rich in beta-carotene) nearby. Try them plain or dipped in hummus or light vinaigrette.
- Limit storage of fruits and vegetables. Once carotenoids are separated from the plant, they begin to break down.
- Check out your local Asian or Latin American grocery store to discover some new vegetables. For fresh, seasonal produce, check out your local farmer's market.
- Avoid overcooking vegetables. While you still get a substantial amount of antioxidants in cooked vegetables, you will get much more if you don't cook them. There are a few exceptions, such as carrots, that actually release more carotenoids if you cook them. If you don't like cooked carrots, try puréeing your raw carrots to release more of their carotenoids.
- Have plenty of tomato products (rich in lycopene): Mix sun-dried tomatoes into bread dough or add them to a veggie sandwich. Top pasta with marinara sauce (and add frozen vegetables, such as spinach or kale, to the sauce as it cooks). Add canned tomatoes or salsa to a bean burrito, or top a veggie burger with ketchup or salsa. Reach for tomato juice to quench your thirst. Or make a quick bruschetta by toasting baguette slices and then topping them with canned, diced tomatoes and a sprinkling of basil.
- For a refreshing start to your day, try a pink grapefruit (rich in lycopene and vitamin C).
- Crush a brazil nut (rich in selenium) on top of your vegetable salad.
- Enjoy beans and whole grains for vitamin E and selenium.
- Add blueberries (rich in vitamin E) to your cereal or fruit smoothie.
- Add barley (rich in vitamin E and selenium) instead of pasta to vegetable soups and stews.
- Add broccoli, cauliflower, or any other of the other cruciferous veggies to stir-fries, soups, stews, and sauces.
- Boost any salad's cancer-fighting potential by adding watercress, kale, cabbage, or collard greens.
- Use rutabagas or turnips in place of potatoes in your favorite potato dish.
- Add fresh garlic to almost any meal.

Recommended Recipes

Fresh Spinach Salad (page 97)
Zippy Yams and Collards (page 108)
Mashed Grains and Cauliflower (page 104)
Mushroom Gravy (page 143)
Summer Fruit Compote (page 132)

To Do This Week

Prepare one meal rich in beta-carotene and another rich in lycopene. This is easy, of course—it is as simple as cooking up some carrots and pouring tomato sauce over your angel hair pasta.

Select your recipes and plan a time that is convenient for you to pick up the ingredients you'll need.

When you enter the grocery store to pick up your ingredients, pause for a moment in the produce aisle. Notice the bright colors and the fact that the same colors tend to show up over and over. Which foods have beta-carotene's distinctive color? That's right—you see it in cantaloupes, sweet potatoes, carrots, and occasionally in other foods.

Which ones have lycopene? It just about jumps out of the tomato bins. And you'll see it in the big watermelon slices and pink grapefruit.

Look at chlorophyll's bright green color almost everywhere in the produce section, and all the various other intense colors. These pigments are not just there to look pretty in your shopping cart. They served to protect the plants, and they will protect you, too.

Also, try preparing any cruciferous vegetable that is new to you, or prepare an old favorite in a new way. For example, if Brussels sprouts always seemed like a punishment instead of a food, try this: Start with frozen petite Brussels sprouts—the smaller they are, the more tender their taste. Steam them until they are soft and tender, then splash on some soy sauce, apple cider vinegar, or balsamic vinegar. You will be amazed. Try the same sort of technique with broccoli, kale, or collards.

If you've never had Swiss chard, it's time to try this wonderful vegetable. A few minutes of steaming turns it into a delightfully tender side dish. Top it with lemon juice. You'll find that the tartness of lemon juice or apple cider vinegar cuts through the faintly bitter taste of many vegetables and makes them truly delectable.

Section 6 References

1. Rock CL, Demark-Wahnefried W. Nutrition and survival after the diagnosis of breast cancer: a review of the evidence. J Clin Oncol 2002;20:3302-16.

2. Murillo G, Mehta RG. Cruciferous vegetables and cancer prevention. Nutr Cancer 2001;41:17-28.

3. Giovannucci E, Rimm EB, Liu Y, Stampfer MJ, Willett WC. A prospective study of tomato products, lycopene, and prostate cancer risk. J Natl Cancer Inst 2002;94:391-8.

4. Saintot M, Matthieu-Daude H, Astre C, Grenier J, Simony-Lafontaine J, Gerber M. Oxidant-antioxidant status in relation to survival among breast cancer patients. Int J Cancer 2002;97:574-9.

5. Chiao JW, Chung FL, Kancherla R, Ahmed T, Mittelman A, Conaway CC. Sulforaphane and its metabolite mediate growth arrest and apoptosis in human prostate cancer cells. Int J Oncol 2002;20:631-6.

6. Bell MC, Crowley-Nowick P, Bradlow HL, et al. Placebo-controlled trial of indole-3-carbinol in the treatment of CIN. Gynecol Oncol 2000;78:123-9.

7. Le Bon AM, Siess MH. Organosulfur compounds from *Allium* and their chemoprevention of cancer. Drug Metabol Drug Interact. 2000;17:51-79.

8. Pinto JT, Lapsia S, Shah A, Santiago H, Kim G. Antiproliferative effects of garlic-derived and other allium related compounds. Adv Exp Med Biol. 2001;492:83-106.

9. Nagourney RA. Garlic: Medicinal food or nutritious medicine. J Medicinal Food 1998;1:13-28.

10. Song K, Milner JA. The influence of heating on the anticancer properties of garlic. J Nutr 2001;131:1054S-57S.

SECTION 7

Immune-Boosting Foods

If you were to look at a sample of your blood under a microscope, you would see an enormous number of red blood cells whose job is to carry oxygen to your body tissues. Here and there among them are white blood cells of various kinds, and they are the key soldiers that make up your immune system. When abnormal cells arise in the body, it is white blood cells' job to recognize and eliminate them.

Some white blood cells are able to engulf and destroy abnormal cells—including cancer cells—as well as viruses, bacteria, and other invaders. Other white blood cells facilitate this process in various ways, for example, by producing *antibodies*, protein molecules that attach to foreign or abnormal cells and flag them for destruction.

The immune system is critically important in fighting cancer. Individual cancer cells can arise in all of us from time to time. Cancer cells can also break free from an existing tumor and spread to other parts of the body. If your immune system is vigilant, it recognizes and destroys cancer cells before they can take hold. So strengthening the immune system is a key strategy in cancer prevention and survival.

Foods That Boost Immunity

Like soldiers anywhere, your immune cells fight more effectively when they are well nourished. Certain nutrients have been shown to be immune boosters.

Beta-carotene. As we saw in Section 6, beta-carotene is an important antioxidant. It also boosts immune function. The best sources are orange and yellow vegetables and fruits, such as carrots, yams, and cantaloupes, as well as green, leafy vegetables. For a detailed list of beta-carotene–rich foods, check the table in Section 6. Research has shown that beta-carotene supplements are not necessarily as safe or effective as food-derived beta-carotene.

The U.S. Government does not have a specific recommended intake for beta-carotene, except to say that 11 milligrams per day for men and 9 milligrams per day for women will give you your daily dose of vitamin A (beta-carotene is converted to vitamin A in the body). Research studies generally use somewhat higher intakes and have shown that the amount of beta-carotene in two large carrots (about 30 milligrams) consumed daily has a measurable immune-boosting effect.[1,2]

Vitamin C. Nobel Laureate Linus Pauling was a strong advocate for vitamin C, and research suggests that, indeed, vitamin C boosts immunity, in addition to its antioxidant abilities. Once again, vegetables and fruits are the preferred sources. Vitamin C-rich foods are listed in Section 6.

The recommended daily intake is only 90 milligrams per day for men and 75 milligrams per day for women. However, some researchers have recommended higher amounts, typically in the form of supplements and usually in the neighborhood of 500 to 2,000 milligrams. There appear to be no adverse effects from these higher doses of vitamin C.

Vitamin E. When it comes to vitamin E, a little is good, but a lot is not necessarily better. Researchers have found that individuals eating vitamin E-rich foods (see tables in Section Six) tend to have improved immunity. But increasing vitamin E intake to high levels through supplements can impair immune function.[3] The best advice appears to be to stick with food sources and avoid vitamin E supplements.

Zinc. The mineral zinc has been promoted for its cold-fighting abilities, and, indeed, it works. However, when it comes to zinc or any other mineral, you want neither too little nor too much, just as we saw with vitamin E.[4] Researchers in New Jersey discovered this fact accidentally.[5] They tested zinc's effects in a group of older men and women. Some were given zinc tablets, while others got placebo tablets that looked and tasted just like zinc. And to make sure that everyone was generally well-nourished, the researchers also asked everyone to take a daily multiple vitamin.

When the researchers later checked their immune function, they found, to their surprise, that *everyone* had an immune boost. You can guess why. The multiple vitamin apparently counteracted a variety of mild nutritional deficiencies, and that improved their immunity. However, the researchers had a second, and more surprising finding: The volunteers taking as little as 15 milligrams of zinc actually had *worse* immune function than those who got placebos. In other words, zinc is an essential nutrient and a helpful immune booster when ingested in minute quantities. But it is easy to go overboard, and excess zinc *interferes* with immune function. The recommended amount of zinc in the daily diet is 8 milligrams for adult women and 11 milligrams for adult men. Here are some good foods that will keep your zinc intake up where it should be, without going too high:

Zinc (mg)

1 serving of most breakfast cereals	3.75
1 Yves Veggie Burger	9.2
½ cup tempeh	1.3
½ cup peas	0.8
½ cup cooked chickpeas	1.3
1 cup soymilk	0.9
2 Tbsp. tahini	1.4
2 Tbsp. wheat germ	2.3

Foods That Interfere with Immunity

In contrast to these healthy immune boosters, some parts of the diet interfere with immunity. Fatty foods, in particular, impair your immune cells' ability to work. Researchers have fed fatty foods to volunteers, dripped fatty intravenous solutions into volunteers' bloodstreams, and mixed fats with cancer cells. In each case, immune strength is noticeably reduced.[6-8] Simply put, your white blood cells don't work very well in an oil slick. While many people avoid animal fats—which is a good idea—they give themselves free rein with vegetable oils. But when it comes to boosting immunity, you'll want to minimize *all* fats and oils. This includes fish oils. Several research studies have suggested that fish oils can interfere with immunity.[9,10]

Fatty foods probably affect white blood cells directly. But they also tend to cause weight gain, and that can further impair immune function.[11] Studies show that overweight individuals are at increased susceptibility to various infections and to certain forms of cancer, especially postmenopausal breast cancer.

Cholesterol also seems to interfere with immunity. In case you are confused about the difference between fat and cholesterol: Fat is visible as a yellow layer under a chicken skin or white streaks marbled through a cut of beef. Cholesterol, on the other hand, resides as tiny particles inside the cell membranes that surround each cell in an animal's body, and *it is primarily in the lean portion.* Essentially all animal products contain cholesterol, while plant products never do.

When researchers add cholesterol to white blood cells in the test tube, it clearly interferes with their ability to function. Because your liver makes all the cholesterol your body needs for normal function, there is no need for any cholesterol in the diet.

Vegetarian Diets and Immunity

Vegetarian diets are typically rich in vitamins. They are low in fat, and vegetarians who also avoid dairy products and eggs (i.e., vegans) have no cholesterol in their diets at all. Vegetarian diets also help people lose excess weight; overweight people switching to a vegetarian diet typically lose about ten percent of their body weight. So, theoretically, vegetarian diets ought to boost immunity.

That theory was put to the test at the German Cancer Research Center. Researchers drew blood samples from a group of vegetarians and compared them to healthy nonvegetarians working at the research center. They separated out a particular type of white blood cell called a *natural killer cell.* As its name implies, it really does shoot first and ask questions later. Natural killer (or NK) cells engulf and destroy cancer cells.

By mixing the volunteers' NK cells with standardized samples of cancer cells, the researchers found that the vegetarians had approximately double the natural killer cell activity, compared to the nonvegetarians.[12]

Your white blood cells don't work very well in an oil slick.

Meal Planning

Here are the keys to an immune-boosting menu:

- Have plenty of vegetables and fruits—five to six servings a day. One serving of vegetables is one-half cup cooked or one cup raw. For fruit, a serving is one small whole fruit or one-half cup chopped fruit.
- Round out your diet with whole grains and legumes (beans, peas, and lentils).
- Take a multiple vitamin each day.
- By avoiding animal products, you'll avoid most fat and all dietary cholesterol.
- By avoiding added oils, you'll keep fat content very low and immunity high.

Recommended Recipes

Spinach Salad with Fruit Flavors (page 99)
Creamy Veggie Curry (page 116) over quinoa
Gingered Melon Wedges (page 130)

Section 7 References

1. Bendich A. Carotenoids and the immune response. J Nutr 1989;119:112-15.

2. Watson RR, Prabhala RH, Plezia PM, Alberts DS. Effect of beta-carotene on lymphocyte subpopulations in elderly humans: evidence for a dose-response relationship. Am J Clin Nutr 1991;53:90-4.

3. Chandra RK. Nutrition and the immune system from birth to old age. Eur J Clin Nutr 2002;56:S73-6.

4. Dardenne M. Zinc and immune function. Eur J Clin Nutr 2002;56:S20-3.

5. Bogden JD, Oleske JM, Lavenhar MA, et al. Effects of one year of supplementation with zinc and other micro-nutrients on cellular immunity in the elderly. J Am Coll Nutr 1990;9:214-25.

6. Hawley HP, Gordon GB. The effects of long chain free fatty acids on human neutrophil function and structure. Lab Invest 1976;34:216-22.

7. Barone J, Hebert JR, Reddy MM. Dietary fat and natural-killer-cell activity. Am J Clin Nutr 1989;50:861-67.

8. Nordenstrom J, Jarstrand C, Wiernik A. Decreased chemotactic and random migration of leukocytes during intralipid infusion. Am J Clin Nutr 1979;32:2416-22.

9. Von Schacky CS, Fischer S, Weber PC. Long-term effect of dietary marine omega-3 fatty acids upon plasma and cellular lipids, platelet function, and eicosanoid formation in humans. J Clin Invest 1985;76:1626-31.

10. Endres S, Ghorbani R, Kelley VE, et al. The effect of dietary supplementation with n-3 polyunsaturated fatty acids on the synthesis of interleukin-1 and tumor necrosis factor by mononuclear cells. N Engl J Med 1989;320:265-71.

11. Lamas O, Marti A, Martinez JA. Obesity and immunocompetence. Eur J Clin Nutr 2002;56:S42-5.

12. Malter M, Schriever G, Eilber U. Natural killer cells, vitamins, and other blood components of vegetarian and omnivorous men. Nutr Cancer 1989;12:271-8.

Maintaining a Healthy Weight

Many studies have shown that slimmer people are less likely to develop cancer. And trimming excess weight may also improve survival after cancer has been diagnosed. Among women with breast cancer, for example, at least 17 different research studies have shown that those who are thinner tend to live longer and have less risk of recurrence.[1]

Researchers have not had to look very hard to find reasons to explain this finding. It has long been known that body fat is like a factory producing estrogens (female sex hormones). What happens is that hormones are produced in the adrenal glands (small organs above each kidney) and are then carried through the bloodstream into body fat. There, fat cells convert these hormones into estrogens.[1] In turn, estrogens fuel breast cancer growth, as we saw in Section 1.

That's not all. Both women and men who have more body fat tend to have less of a protein compound called *sex hormone binding globulin* (SHBG) in their blood. SHBG's job is to bind estrogen and testosterone, keeping these hormones inactive and unable to promote cancer. If overweight people have less SHBG, it means that more of their hormones are not reined in. They travel freely in the bloodstream, increasing the risk that cancer will start or, if it has started, will spread to other parts of the body.

Excess weight may also reduce immune defenses. Researchers have shown that overweight people are more likely to show other signs of flagging immunity, such as recurrent infections. Poor immune defenses could mean they are less able to combat cancer cells that may arise.[2]

Body fat is like an estrogen factory. Fat cells convert other hormones into estrogens.

Trimming Down the Healthy Way

So how do we slim down? The first key is to focus not on *how much* you eat, but on *what* you eat. It is natural for people seeking to lose weight to skip meals and eat tiny portions. But doing so over even a few weeks tends to slow down your body's calorie-burning speed, making it harder and harder to lose weight. And cutting back on portions can make hunger get out of control, leading to binges and rebound weight gain.

Instead, focus on healthful foods that are naturally modest in calories. The best advice is to build your menu from the New Four Food Groups that we met in Section 1. Vegetables, fruits, beans, and whole grains are nearly always lower in calories than typical meats, dairy products, eggs, and fried foods. This is partly because they are usually very low in fat. Ounce for ounce, fat has more than twice the calories of carbohydrate or protein. In addition, plant-based foods are so high in fiber, they tend to fill you up before you've taken in too many calories. Studies show that every 14 grams of fiber in your daily diet reduces your calorie intake by about ten percent.[3]

So, build your diet from the New Four Food Groups. At the same time, avoid animal products and keep vegetable oils to an absolute minimum. In the process, you'll eliminate all animal fat and fiber-depleted foods and dramatically cut your fat intake.

Several studies by the research team at the Physicians Committee for Responsible Medicine have shown that simply using the New Four Food Groups while avoiding animal products and keeping oils to a minimum leads to a weight loss of about one pound per week—week after week after week—*even if you don't exercise.* For example, in a study of 59 postmenopausal women, the diet change caused participants to lose an average of 13 pounds in 14 weeks. The same effect was seen in young women.[4] And in a study of individuals with type 2 diabetes, participants lost an average of 16 pounds in just 12 weeks.[5]

Many other research studies have reached similar conclusions. You can focus on the type of food you eat—not the amount—and lose weight naturally and safely.

Of course, a slimmer body is not the only benefit of this sort of healthy menu. Low-fat vegetarian and vegan diets have been used to reverse heart disease, bring diabetes under control, lower blood pressure, reduce menstrual and premenstrual symptoms, and achieve many other health goals.[4–8]

Avoid Risky Diets

Some fad diets have had on-again, off-again popularity but are very unhealthy over the long run. For example, low-carbohydrate, high-protein diets eliminate bread, pasta, beans, rice, starchy vegetables, and other carbohydrate-rich foods and focus instead on meat and eggs. There are several things wrong with such diets.

First, controlled tests show that these diets cause weight loss that is no quicker than that associated with old-fashioned low-calorie diets or with healthy low-fat, vegan diets. All of these regimens lead to a weight reduction of about one pound per week.

Second, when people lose weight with high-protein diets, it is simply because they are eliminating so many other foods that their overall calorie intake drops. If overall calorie intake doesn't drop, they don't lose weight.

Most importantly, high-protein diets are linked to significant problems. Researchers have found that people on these diets lose large amounts of calcium in their urine, and the loss is caused by the massive amounts of protein they are consuming.[9] Animal protein tends to leach calcium from the bones and send it through the kidneys into the urine. Over the long run, that can lead to osteoporosis.

As we saw in Section 4, meaty diets are linked to higher risk of colon

Studies show that every 14 grams of fiber in your daily diet reduces your calorie intake by about ten percent.

cancer.[10,11] And high-fat diets in general are linked to poorer survival in individuals diagnosed with cancer.

For individuals battling serious illness—and for anyone else—it is a very good idea to lose excess weight, and it is important to do so in as healthful a way as possible.

Exercise

Exercise burns calories, boosts your metabolism, and helps reduce the stresses that can lead to binge eating. But don't jump into a vigorous regimen too quickly. If you're over 40, significantly overweight, or dealing with any serious medical condition, you should check with your doctor before greatly increasing your physical activity.

When you start an exercise program, it pays to begin slowly. For most people, a brisk walk every day for half an hour—or three times per week for an hour—is a good way to begin.

If you are unable to exercise because of joint problems, cardiac limitations, or any other reason, you'll be glad to know that a low-fat diet based on the New Four Food Groups typically brings weight loss even when people do not exercise. Yes, exercise is a good thing, but it is not essential for weight loss.

Weight-Loss Keys

To summarize, here are the keys to healthy weight loss:
- Build your diet from the New Four Food Groups: vegetables, fruits, beans, and whole grains.
- Avoid animal products and added vegetable oils.
- Add any common multiple vitamin as a source of vitamin B_{12}.
- There are not many fatty plant foods, but it is good to minimize the ones there are—nuts, seeds, avocados, olives, and some soy products.
- Go high-fiber, having plenty of vegetables, fruits, and bean dishes in as natural and unprocessed a state as possible. Choose high-fiber grains, such as brown rice instead of white rice and whole grain bread instead of white bread.
- If your doctor gives you the green light for regular physical activity, be sure to add exercise to your routine. Start slowly. Brisk walking for a half-hour daily or an hour three times a week is a good way to begin. Then gradually increase your regimen.

Meal Planning

If you're aiming to knock off some pounds, this is a great time for a new focus on high-fiber foods. They tend to be very low in fat, so they won't add many calories. And they will fill you up, so you're less likely to overdo it.

If you were to include high-fiber foods at breakfast, lunch, and dinner, what would they be? Here are a few ideas, but think about ones that are most appealing to you:

Breakfast: Old-fashioned oatmeal is a natural choice. A bowl of strawberries or half a cantaloupe will add fiber, too. And, while it might sound a bit odd at first, a serving of chickpeas at breakfast provides plenty of protein and fiber, with very little fat—try it; you'll like it. Whole-grain breads and bran cereals with low-fat soymilk or rice milk will also give you plenty of fiber.

Lunch: Start with salads loaded with fresh vegetables, beans, and low-fat salad dressing. For a hearty lunch, baked beans, lentil soup, or bean burritos are unbeatable. Or try hummus tucked into whole-wheat pita bread with grated carrots, sprouts, and cucumbers, or spread low-fat black bean dip into a whole-wheat tortilla and wrap it with peppers, tomatoes, and lettuce. A side of steamed green vegetables is always a great addition. And, if your tastes call for fresh fruit, a couple of pears or apples will give you loads of fiber with very few calories.

Dinner: For dinner, there are endless choices: vegetable stir-fry over brown rice, a chunky vegetable chili, lentil curry, vegetable fajitas loaded with fat-free "refried" beans and sautéed vegetables, or vegetable lasagna layered with tomato sauce, crumbled tofu, spinach, mushrooms, and cheesy nutritional yeast in place of the usual fatty meat and cheese. Or keep it simple and enjoy whole wheat pasta with a vegetable-heavy marinara sauce. For dessert, try fresh fruit or a fruit sorbet.

Recommended Recipes

Veggies in a Blanket (page 85)
Sesame Bok Choy and Carrot Stir-Fry (page 122)
Lentil and Artichoke Stew (page 89)

Section 8 References

1. Rock CL, Demark-Wahnefried W. Nutrition and survival after the diagnosis of breast cancer: a review of the evidence. J Clin Oncol 2002;20:3302-16.

2. Lamas O, Marti A, Martinez JA. Obesity and immunocompetence. Eur J Clin Nutr 2002;56 (Suppl 1):S42-5.

3. Howarth NC, Saltzman E, Roberts SB. Dietary fiber and weight regulation. Nutr Rev 2001;59:129-39.

4. Barnard ND, Scialli AR, Hurlock D, Bertron P. Diet and sex-hormone binding globulin, dysmenorrhea, and premenstrual symptoms. Obstet Gynecol 2000a;95:245-50.

5. Nicholson AS, Sklar M, Barnard ND, Gore S, Sullivan R, Browning S. Toward improved management of NIDDM: a randomized, controlled, pilot intervention using a low-fat, vegetarian diet. Prev Med 1999;29:87-91.

6. Ornish D, Brown SE, Scherwitz LW, Billings JH, Armstrong WT, Ports TA. Can lifestyle changes reverse coronary heart disease? Lancet 1990;336:129-33.

7. Barnard ND, Nicholson A, Howard JL. The medical costs attributable to meat consumption. Prev Med 1995;24:646-55.

8. Barnard ND, Scialli AR, Bertron P, Hurlock D, Edmonds K, Talev L. Effectiveness of a low-fat, vegetarian diet in altering serum lipids in healthy premenopausal women. Am J Cardiol 2000b;85:969-72.

9. Reddy ST, Wang CY, Sakhaee K, Brinkley L, Pak CY. Effect of low-carbohydrate high-protein diets on acid-base balance, stone-forming propensity, and calcium metabolism. Am J Kidney Dis 2002;40:265-74.

10. Willett WC, Stampfer MJ, Colditz GA, Rosner BA, Speizer FE. Relation of meat, fat, and fiber intake to the risk of colon cancer in a prospective study among women. N Engl J Med 1990;323:1664-72.

11. Giovannucci E, Rimm EB, Stampfer MJ, Colditz GA, Ascherio A, Willett WC. Intake of fat, meat, and fiber in relation to risk of colon cancer in men. Cancer Res 1994;54:2390-7.

Nutrition Basics

Let's define the basic terms nutritionists use in planning out healthy diets. What exactly do we mean when we talk about carbohydrate, protein, and fat? What are they for, and how much (or how little) of each should we be getting each day?

Good nutrition means getting these nutrients, along with fiber, vitamins, and minerals, not only in the right amounts, but also the right form. This section will help you understand the basics of the macronutrients (carbohydrate, protein, and fat) and fiber —why we need them, and what the most healthful choices are.

Carbohydrate

Carbohydrate is the main source of calories in a healthy diet. It is the primary fuel source for the brain and muscles and helps maintain nervous system function. Normally, your body stores a bit of carbohydrate in your muscles and liver as *glycogen*, which acts as a reserve energy source. Liver glycogen maintains blood glucose levels, but it is depleted within 18 hours if no carbohydrate is consumed. When that happens, your body can make carbohydrate from amino acids that are drawn from your muscles, but that means that your muscle mass will dwindle. Low-carbohydrate diets prevent the complete breakdown of fat, which leads to the production of ketones. During this time, the body goes to its fat stores for energy. People who are using ketones for energy (versus carbohydrates) experience bad breath, headaches, and fatigue. Plus, since our brain works exclusively on glucose, people not consuming enough carbohydrate may experience decreased mental functioning.

There are two types of carbohydrate: simple and complex. *Simple carbohydrates*, or sweets, are the quickest source of energy because they lack bulk (fiber). Because simple carbohydrates turn into glucose so quickly in our bloodstreams, they can be useful for someone having a hypoglycemic episode. However, for the most part, simple carbohydrates are discouraged because they are low in fiber, high in sugar, and low in vitamins and minerals, and they do not signal our brains that we've had enough to eat. You may have noticed that you're much more satiated with a snack of fat-free popcorn than you are with sugar candies. Some simple carbohydrates:

- Table sugar
- Brown sugar
- Fruit juices
- Honey
- Jams, jellies
- Maple syrup
- Molasses

Complex carbohydrates, on the other hand, are rich in fiber, more satisfying, more health-promoting because they are high in vitamins and minerals, important for proper digestion and elimination, and important for colon health and proper elimination. Some complex carbohydrates:

- Vegetables   • Fruits   • Whole grains   • Potatoes   • Beans

Approximately 55–75 percent of daily calories should come from carbohydrate. For an average adult, that works out to about 275–375 grams of carbohydrate per day.

Fiber

Fiber is only found in plant foods. This is why vegetarians, particularly vegans, often have a high fiber intake. Fiber provides us with many benefits, including cancer prevention, as we saw in Section 2. Fiber intake is one of the reasons vegetarians have significantly lower rates of cancer, heart disease, and diabetes and are usually slimmer than other people. Fiber helps you to "fill up" so that you don't "fill out."

There are two types of fiber: insoluble and soluble. It's important to have both insoluble and soluble fiber in your diet. Most foods contain a mixture of both fibers, and the two types are not usually differentiated on the food label.

Insoluble fiber is not readily metabolized by the bacteria in your intestinal tract and does not readily dissolve in water. It increases fecal bulk and decreases intestinal transit time. All plants, especially vegetables, wheat, wheat bran, rye, and rice are rich in insoluble fiber.

Soluble fiber dissolves or swells when it is put into water and is readily metabolized by intestinal bacteria. It has been shown to help lower cholesterol levels and slow down gastric emptying time (thus keeping you full longer). Beans, fruits, and oats are especially good sources of soluble fiber. Other examples of soluble fibers include guar gum and locust bean gum—these are found in salad dressings and jams.

Most health authorities recommended fiber intake in the range of 25–35 grams per day as a minimal goal, and, optimally, your goal should be about 40 grams. The average American eats 14–15 grams a day, and vegetarians get two to three times that amount.

Here are the fiber contents of some common foods:

- 5 grams of fiber per serving: beans, pear with skin, raspberries, whole-wheat spaghetti, bran cereals
- 3 grams of fiber per serving: apple with skin, blueberries, corn, orange, potato with skin, strawberries
- 2 grams of fiber per serving: banana, broccoli, mango, mixed veggies, oatmeal, whole-grain bread, peach

Increase your fiber intake slowly, and increase water intake as well.

Protein

Protein is needed to build and repair muscles, bones, skin, and blood; regulate hormones and enzymes; and help fight infection and heal wounds. It is also an integral part of genes and chromosomes.

The building blocks of protein are called *amino acids*. The body can synthesize some amino acids; others must be ingested from food. Of the 20 or so different amino acids in the food we eat, our bodies can make 11. The 9 remaining amino acids are called *essential amino acids*—that is, the body cannot produce them, and they must be obtained from the diet.

It is remarkably easy to get enough protein. A variety of grains, legumes, and vegetables can provide all of the essential amino acids our bodies require. It was once thought that, to get their full protein value, various plant foods had to be consumed together, a practice known as protein combining or protein complementing. However, researchers have found that intentional combining is not necessary. As long as the diet contains a variety of grains, legumes, and vegetables, protein needs are easily met.

Approximately 10–15 percent of daily calories should come from protein—protein needs depend on body weight and increase with activity level and body stress (such as tissue repair, medical treatments, etc.). Like carbohydrates, there are 4 calories in 1 gram of protein. All foods except pure fats, sugars, and fruits contain protein. The Recommended Dietary Allowance (RDA) for protein for the average, sedentary adult is only 0.8 grams per kilogram of body weight, with protein needs increasing only slightly with more activity. To find out your average individual need, simply perform the following calculation:

- Body weight (in pounds) × 0.36 = recommended protein intake (in grams)
- Example:
  - A person who weighs 150 lbs. needs 54 grams of protein per day.
  - What does 54 grams of protein taste like?
    - 1 bowl of Raisin Bran and 1 cup soymilk (12 grams) +
    - 1 veggie burger and whole-wheat bun (20 grams) +
    - 1 cup pasta with 1 cup assorted vegetables and beans (22 grams) = 54 grams of protein.

The most protein-rich plant foods are listed in the table on the following page. Of all plant foods, legumes (beans, peas, and lentils) are more nutrient dense and easily supply a substantial amount of protein. Most varieties of legumes are about 25 percent protein and yield approximately 15 grams of protein per cup. But don't think that beans have a patent on protein. Wheat noodles contain substantial amounts; some varieties have about 10 grams of protein in every two ounces of dry pasta, and that's before you figure in any toppings.

Higher-Protein Plant Foods (serving size: 1 cup)	Calories	Protein (g)	Fat (g)
LEGUMES (cooked)			
Baked beans (vegetarian)	235	12.2	1.1
Black beans	227	15.2	0.9
Chickpeas	285	11.9	2.7
Kidney beans	225	15.4	0.9
Lentils	231	17.9	0.7
Pinto beans	235	14.0	0.9
Split peas	231	16.4	0.8
SOYBEAN PRODUCTS			
Soymilk	140	10.0	4.0
Tempeh burger (1 burger)	110	12.5	3.2
Textured vegetable protein (prepared)	120	22.0	0.2
Tofu (firm)	366	39.8	22.0
BREAKFAST CEREALS			
All Bran	213	12.0	1.5
Grape-Nuts	416	12.4	0.4

Fat

Fat is the most concentrated source of calories in the food you eat. Any sort of fat—chicken fat, fish fat, beef fat, or vegetable oil—has 9 calories per gram, more than twice the calorie content of carbohydrate or protein. Most health authorities recommend that fat intake not exceed 30 percent of your calories. This means that a person consuming 2000 calories per day should have less than 60 grams of fat per day.

However, research has shown that the lower your fat intake, the better your chances of warding off heart disease and cancer and keeping your waistline slim.

Fats are made up of a combination of *fatty acids*, which can be *monounsaturated*, *polyunsaturated*, or *saturated*. All fats contain some of each of these three, but health authorities have long recommended minimizing saturated fats because of their tendency to raise cholesterol levels. Animal products are generally very high in saturated fatty acids whereas vegetable oils are generally much lower in this type of fat. There are a few exceptions: coconut oil, palm oil, and palm kernel oil are quite high in saturated fat.

Foods high in monounsaturated fatty acids and low in saturated fatty acids include:
- Olives, olive oil
- Almonds, almond oil, almond butter
- Canola oil (also called rapeseed oil)

- Hazelnuts (also called filberts)
- Peanuts, peanut oil, natural peanut butter
- Avocados

Foods high in polyunsaturated fatty acids include:
- Sesame seeds, sesame oil, sesame butter
- Sunflower seeds, sunflower oil
- Safflower oil
- Corn oil
- Walnuts, walnut oil
- Soybeans and soy products (tofu, tempeh, TVP)
- Flax seeds, flax seed oil

Foods high in saturated fatty acids include:
- Foods of animal origin (beef, pork, lamb, poultry, eggs, milk, butter, cheese, sour cream, etc.)
- Tropical oils, such as coconut, palm, and palm kernel oils
- Chocolate, cocoa butter

Fat is necessary for structure and maintenance of cells and hormones, healthy skin and hair, and the metabolism of fat-soluble vitamins (A, D, E, and K). As long as we consume enough calories, we can synthesize fat from surplus protein and carbohydrates. However, there are two *essential fatty acids* that we need to obtain from our diet. They are alpha-linolenic acid (an omega-3 fatty acid) and alpha-linoleic acid (an omega-6 fatty acid). Both are important in the normal functioning of all tissues of the body. Deficiencies are responsible for a host of symptoms and disorders, including abnormalities in the liver and kidney, changes in the blood, reduced growth rates, decreased immune function, and skin changes, including dryness and scaliness. Adequate intake of the essential fatty acids results in numerous health benefits. Prevention of atherosclerosis, reduced incidence of heart disease and stroke, and relief from the symptoms associated with ulcerative colitis, menstrual pain, and joint pain have also been documented.

Most people consume too many omega-6 fatty acids and too few omega-3 fatty acids. It's important to maintain a balance of these two. Omega-6 fatty acids are present in higher concentrations in many foods, whereas omega-3 fatty acids are not as widespread. Beans, vegetables, fruits, and vegetables do contain omega-3 fatty acids, but the most concentrated plant sources include canola oil, flaxseeds, wheat germ, soybeans, and walnuts.

Scientific Findings on Diet's Effect on Cancer Survival

Foods and Breast Cancer Survival

Healthful diets not only help prevent cancer; they also improve survival when cancer has been diagnosed. The first clues that foods might affect the course of breast cancer came from studies of women in Japan in the early 1960s. Compared to Western women, Japanese women were much less likely to develop the disease and much more likely to survive it if it occurred.[1] Over the next several decades, researchers have followed up on these observations to try to clarify what is the best diet for cancer survival. Although this work is still in its early stages, important information has already come to light.

One of the best-established factors affecting breast cancer survival is body weight. Women with breast cancer who are near their ideal body weight at the time of diagnosis are more likely to survive than are women with higher body weights.[2] And although weight gain often occurs after diagnosis, studies suggest that women who avoid weight gain after diagnosis tend to have longer disease-free survival.[2]

The link between lower body weight and better survival may relate to estrogens, female sex hormones that can encourage the growth of cancer cells. In essence, body fat acts like an estrogen factory, producing estrogens from other compounds coming from the adrenal glands (small organs situated atop each kidney). As a result, women with more body fat tend to have higher amounts of estrogens circulating in their blood, compared to leaner women.

Reduced Fat Intake

Specific dietary factors appear to play key roles in cancer survival. First, two studies of women diagnosed with breast cancer showed that those who had been consuming less fat prior to diagnosis generally had smaller tumors with less evidence of cancer spread, compared to women whose diets had included more fatty foods.[3,4] One of these studies identified benefits among premenopausal women; the other, among postmenopausal women.

Studies that have followed women for several years after diagnosis have generally found that those with less fatty diets prior to diagnosis live longer than other women. In one of the first such studies, researchers at the State University of New York in Buffalo, N.Y., found that women with advanced cancer had a 40 percent increased risk of dying at any point in time for every 1,000 grams of fat they consumed per month.[5] Note that this does not mean a person's risk of dying is 40 percent. It means that, if a person's diet contains an extra 1,000 grams of fat per month at the time of diagnosis, that person's risk of dying is 40 percent higher than it would otherwise have been. There is, of course, tremendous variation from one woman to another, so this figure is simply an overall observation drawn from the group of participants. To make this more concrete: The difference between a typical American diet and a low-fat, vegan diet is approximately 1,000–1,500 grams of fat per month, which corresponds to a 40–60 percent difference in mortality risk at any point in time.

Other studies found much the same thing—fatty diets are associated with increased risk, and that is particularly true for saturated fat, the kind that is common in meat, dairy products, eggs, and chocolate.[6–9] Some studies have failed to confirm the dangers of fatty diets.[10–13] However, most evidence indicates that women consuming less fat tend to do better after diagnosis, including a new study done by the National Cancer Institute (NCI). This study followed nearly 2,500 post-menopausal women with breast cancer for five years after their standard surgery and cancer treatments. Researchers instructed some of them to continue their regular diets while the rest were put on a low-fat diet. The women continuing their usual diets consumed an average of 51.3 grams of fat per day, which is still lower than the average American's fat, while the low-fat group averaged 33.3 grams per day—slightly more than in a typical vegetarian diet. After five years, 12.4 percent of the women eating their usual diet had cancer recurrences compared to only 9.8 percent of the low-fat diet group, a 24 percent reduction in recurrence.[14]

Why should a low fat intake improve survival? For starters, low-fat diets tend to be modest in calories, since fats and oils are the densest source of calories of any food we consume. In fact, some investigators believe that the main problem with fatty diets is simply their high calorie content. In addition, women who eat less fat tend to have less estrogen coursing through their veins (independent of the difference in their body weight). They may also have stronger immune defenses that can help them fight cancer cells.

Increased Vegetables and Fruits

Some evidence suggests that women whose diets are richer in vegetables and fruits tend to survive longer.[2,15] In a study of 103 women in Australia followed for six years after they were diagnosed with breast cancer, those who consumed the most fruits and vegetables rich in beta-carotene or vitamin C had the best chance for survival. The researchers divided the group into thirds based on how much beta-carotene they got each day in the foods they chose. It turned out that in the group getting the least beta-carotene, there were twelve deaths over the next six years. In the middle group, there were eight deaths, and in the high–beta-carotene group, there was only one death.[16]

In the digestive tract, beta-carotene in converted to vitamin A. In turn, vitamin A is converted to a compound called retinoic acid, which has a demonstrable anti-cancer effect on cells in test-tube studies.[16] A Swedish study found much the same thing: Among women with breast cancer, those consuming more vitamin A were more likely to have estrogen receptor–rich tumors, a good prognostic sign.[17]

The Australian researchers also analyzed their data in another way, looking simply at how much fruit of any kind the women had been eating, including both beta-carotene–rich fruits and other varieties, such as apples, bananas, berries, grapes, and dried fruits. The same sort of pattern emerged. In the group eating the least fruit, there were twelve deaths; in the middle group, there were six deaths; and in the group consuming the most fruit, there were only three deaths.[16]

Similarly, a study of Canadian women with breast cancer found that those getting the most beta-carotene and vitamin C had significantly better survival odds.[8] The benefit was dose related, meaning the more of these helpful nutrients they got, the better they did. Those who got more than 5 milligrams of beta-carotene per day had double the likelihood of survival, compared to women who got less than 2 milligrams. To see what this means on your plate: There are about 5 milligrams of beta-carotene in half a medium carrot or one-fourth cup of cooked sweet potato.

For vitamin C, those getting more than 200 milligrams each day had roughly double the survival odds, compared to those getting less than about 100 milligrams per day. In practical terms, an orange has about 60 milligrams of vitamin C, and a one-cup serving of broccoli or other green vegetables has about 80.[8]

Vitamin E may have the opposite effect. In one study, women with breast cancer consuming larger amounts of vitamin E had poorer survival. Every one-milligram increase in daily vitamin E intake was associated with approximately a 15 to 20 percent increased risk of treatment failure.[7]

Increased Fiber

Fiber is essential to the body's ability to eliminate excess estrogens. As the liver filters estrogens from the blood, it sends them through the bile duct into the intestinal tract, where fiber soaks them up and carries them out of the body. A study in Sweden found that women with higher fiber intake at the time of breast cancer diagnosis were more likely to have smaller tumors, compared to women with lower fiber intake.[17] The amount consumed was not particularly high. Those women with larger tumors (greater than 20 millimeters) averaged 16 grams of fiber per day, compared to 19 grams for women with smaller tumors. Most authorities recommend fiber intake of at least 30 grams daily, and an optimal intake is probably over 40 grams.

Combined Diet Effects

These dietary factors tend to work together. A diet that is higher in fruits and vegetables will also tend to be high in fiber and low in fat. In turn, women who eat such diets tend to be slimmer than other women, avoiding the risks of overweight. One study suggested that there may be a measurable benefit of these combined effects. Researchers at Mt. Sinai Medical Center in New York found that women with breast cancer who were slimmer tended to live longer, and those who had lower cholesterol levels also lived longer. But the women at greatest risk of dying were those who were overweight *and* had high cholesterol levels.[18]

Putting Diet Changes to the Test

The findings described above were generally made by studying the diets of women at the time they were diagnosed with cancer. Generally speaking, women who have been eating fewer fatty foods, more fiber, and more vegetables and fruits at the time of diagnosis live longer and are less likely to have a recurrence. However, it has not yet been proven that changing to a low-fat diet that is loaded with fruits and vegetables after diagnosis will put the brakes on cancer as effectively as having habitually followed such a diet since long before the disease occurred. Studies are now underway to test exactly that.

The Women's Intervention Nutrition Study (WINS) tests a low-fat diet deriving 15 percent of calories from fat in 2,500 postmenopausal women with breast cancer. In the Women's Healthy Eating and Living (WHEL) study, 3,109 pre- and postmenopausal women with breast cancer will be included in a test of a diet rich in fruits and vegetables. The study's daily diet guidelines include five vegetable servings, 16 ounces of vegetable juice, three fruit servings, 30 grams of dietary fiber, and no more than 15–20 percent of calories from fat.[2,19]

One danger in large clinical trials is that their dietary recommendations are sometimes watered down based on the belief that participants will not be willing to make more extensive diet changes. Nonetheless, such studies are important tests of the diets they do prescribe.

Exercise

Exercise may also improve breast cancer survival. A new study published in the *Journal of the American Medical Association* concluded that physical activity after breast cancer diagnosis may reduce a woman's risk of death from this disease. In this study, the greatest benefit was shown in women who exercised the equivalent of walking at an average pace for 3 to 5 hours per week.[20]

Foods and Breast Cancer Survival References

1. Wynder EL, Kajitani T, Kuno J, Lucas JC Jr, DePalo A, Farrow J. A comparison of survival rates between American and Japanese patients with breast cancer. Surg Gynecol Obstet 1963;117:196-200.

2. Rock CL, Demark-Wahnefried W. Nutrition and survival after the diagnosis of breast cancer: a review of the evidence. J Clin Oncol 2002;20:3302-16.

3. Verreault R, Brisson J, Deschenes L, Naud F, Meyer F, Belanger L. Dietary fat in relation to prognostic indicators in breast cancer. J Natl Cancer Inst 1988;80:819-25.

4. Hebert JR, Toporoff E. Dietary exposures and other factors of possible prognostic significance in relation to tumour size and nodal involvement in early-stage breast cancer. Int J Epidemiol 1989;18:518-26.

5. Gregorio DI, Emrich LJ, Graham S, Marshall JR, Nemoto T. Dietary fat consumption and survival among women with breast cancer. J Natl Cancer Inst 1985 Jul;75(1):37-41.

6. Nomura A, Le Marchand L, Kolonel LN, Hankin JH. The effect of dietary fat on breast cancer survival among Caucasian and Japanese women in Hawaii. Breast Cancer Research and Treatment 1991;18:S135-41.

7. Holm LE, Nordevang E, Hjalmar ML, Lidbrink E, Callmer E, Nilsson B. Treatment failure and dietary habits in women with breast cancer. J Natl Cancer Inst 1993;85:32-6.

8. Jain M, Miller AB, To T. Premorbid diet and the prognosis of women with breast cancer. J Natl Cancer Inst 1994;86:1390-7.

9. Zhang S, Folsom AR, Sellers TA, Kushi LH, Potter JD. Better breast cancer survival for postmenopausal women who are less overweight and eat less fat. Cancer 1995;76:275-83.

10. Rohan TE, Hiller JE, McMichael AJ. Dietary factors and survival from breast cancer. Nutr Cancer 1993;20:167-77.

11. Kyogoku S, Hirohata T, Nomura Y, Shigematsu T, Takeshita S, Hirohata I. Diet and prognosis of breast cancer. Nutr Cancer 1992;17:271-7.

12. Newman SC, Miller AB, Howe GR. A study of the effect of weight and dietary fat on breast cancer survival time. Am J Epidemiol 1986;123:767-74.

13. Ewertz M, Gillanders S, Meyer L, Zedeler K. Survival of breast cancer patients in relation to factors which affect risk of developing breast cancer. Int J Cancer 1991;49:526-530.

14. Chlebowski RT. Dietary fat reduction in postmenopausal women with primary breast cancer: Phase III Women's Intervention Nutrition Study (WINS). Paper presented at: American Society of Clinical Oncology Annual Meeting; May 16, 2005; Torrance, CA.

15. Murillo G, Mehta RG. Cruciferous vegetables and cancer prevention. Nutr Cancer 2001;41:17-28.

16. Ingram D. Diet and subsequent survival in women with breast cancer. Br J Cancer 1994;69:592-5.

17. Holm LE, Callmer E, Hjalmar ML, Lidbrink E, Nilsson B, Skoog L. Dietary habits and prognostic factors in breast cancer. J Natl Cancer Inst 1989;81:1218-23.

18. Tartter PI, Papatestas AE, Ioannovich J, Mulvihill MN, Lesnick G, Aufses AH. Cholesterol and obesity as prognostic factors in breast cancer. Cancer 1981;47:2222-7.

19. Pierce JP, Faerber S, Wright FA, et al. A randomized trial of the effect of a plant-based dietary pattern on additional breast cancer events and survival: the Women's Healthy Eating and Living (WHEL) Study. Contr Clin Trials 2002;23:728-56.

20. Holmes MD, Chen WY, Feskanich D, Kroenke CH, Colditz GA. Physical activity and survival after breast cancer diagnosis. JAMA. 2005 May 25;293(20):2479-86.

Foods and Prostate Cancer Survival

Many research studies have shown how foods affect the risk of developing prostate cancer. Vegetables and fruits reduce the risk, while dairy products and fatty foods appear to increase it.

But what about *after* prostate cancer has been diagnosed? Will a change in eating habits help a man beat the disease? More research is needed, but evidence already available suggests that, whatever other treatments a man may undergo, changes in his diet might well save his life.

The first clues that diet could make a big difference in survival emerged from international comparisons in the 1970s. A man in Hong Kong, where diets are rich in rice and vegetables, is half as likely to have cancerous cells in his prostate, compared to a man in Sweden, where diets are high in dairy products and meat. But if cancer happens to strike, a man in Hong Kong is *eight times more likely to survive it*, compared to his Swedish counterpart.[1] In other words, it appears that the same sort of dietary habits that reduce the risk of cancer also slow its progress if it occurs.

Why would diet changes help? One explanation relates to *insulin-like growth factor* (IGF-I), a substance in the bloodstream that is a powerful stimulus for cancer cell growth. Men following plant-based diets have lower IGF-I levels than other men, while dairy products tend to drive IGF-I levels up. Men following low-fat diets also have slightly lower testosterone and estrogen levels and higher levels of a protein called sex hormone binding globulin, which binds and temporarily inactivates testosterone and estrogen. The net effect is a drop in the biochemical factors that stimulate cancer growth.

Putting Diet to the Test

The first prospective studies of diet's potential benefits were purely observational. In 1999, researchers in Québec City reported their findings after following 384 men with prostate cancer over a five-year period. It turned out that those who consumed the most saturated fat—the kind particularly prevalent in meats and dairy products—had three times the risk of dying from the disease, compared to those with the lowest saturated fat intake. Increased risk was also found with higher intakes of total and monounsaturated fat, but these increases were not significant.[2]

The following year, researchers in Toronto and Vancouver reported the results of a study of 263 men with prostate cancer. After adjustment for clinical stage, tumor grade, and other factors, men who consumed the most monounsaturated fat (the type that is abundant in olive and canola oils) lived longest. Their risk of dying was 70 percent lower, compared to those with the lowest intake of monounsaturates. The study also found increased risk from animal fat and saturated fat intake, although these latter findings were not strong enough to reach statistical significance.[3]

Using a Vegan Diet

Dean Ornish, M.D., who had already demonstrated the benefits of a low-fat, vegetarian diet for heart patients (finding that it reversed heart disease in 82 percent of research participants), decided to put a similar program to the test for prostate cancer.[4] The 93 volunteers were men with early-stage cancer who were able to defer treatment, at least for the moment, because they were keeping a careful watch on their prostate-specific antigen (PSA, an index of cancer spread) levels, a strategy known as "watchful waiting." Typically, PSA levels slowly rise, and eventually treatment (e.g., surgery) may be required. Dr. Ornish randomly assigned half the men to their usual care (the control group) and the remaining half to a low-fat, vegan diet, along with moderate aerobic exercise and stress management. In the experimental vegan group, PSA levels decreased by 4 percent after one year, while PSA levels rose by 6 percent in the control group. Six of the men in the control group needed treatment during the one-year study period because their prostate cancer was progressing whereas no one in the experimental group needed treatment during the study period.

Using Diet Against Recurrent Cancer

Dr. Ornish's approach is extremely promising for men with early disease. But what about advanced cancer? Evidence suggests that diet changes can still play a vital role. Two studies have used special diets in men who had previously been operated on for prostate cancer but who had experienced recurrences of their disease. Using a macrobiotic diet emphasizing whole grains, vegetables, and legumes while avoiding dairy products and most meats, nine men with prostate cancer had an average survival of 228 months, compared to 72 months for a matched group of men receiving no special diet.[5]

A study at the University of Massachusetts tested the benefits of a diet change in ten men with prostate cancer that had recurred after surgery. The diet was based on whole grains, legumes, green and yellow vegetables, seeds, soy products, and fruit, and the men were also instructed in stress-reduction techniques. To measure the program's effect, researchers tracked how long it took for the patients' PSA levels to double—the longer the PSA doubling time, the slower the cancer is spreading. Before the study began, the average PSA doubling time was 6.5 months. But after four months in the program, it had slowed to 17.7 months, an encouraging finding. In three of the men, PSA levels actually fell.[6]

An additional survival study is underway at Memorial Sloan-Kettering Cancer Center in New York.[7] And at the University of California at Los Angeles, two studies are in progress:[8] In the first, men with prostate cancer who have elected for "watchful waiting" are randomly assigned to a "Western diet" or a low-fat, high-fiber diet, and serum growth factors and biomarkers are followed. In the second study, men scheduled for radical prostatectomy are given green tea, black tea, or green tea extract prior to surgery, and their prostate tissue is examined for the effects of these treatments. In 2003, an additional pre-prostatectomy study began, studying the effect of a low-fat diet.

Cancer-Fighting Power You Can See

In 2002, researchers at the University of California at Los Angeles reported a series of unusual experiments that demonstrated the power of diet and exercise. They drew blood samples from a group of eight men who had been following a low-fat diet and exercising regularly for several years. They also drew blood samples from overweight men who were not following the diet and exercise program. They added portions of each man's blood serum to test tubes containing standardized prostate cancer cells. Serum from men on the low-fat diet and exercise program slowed cancer cell growth by 49 percent, compared to serum from the other men. How could this be? Differences in testosterone, estrogen, and insulin account for part of the effect, but other changes in the blood exert additional effects the researchers have not yet teased out.[9] The research team also found that a man's serum shows demonstrable cancer-inhibiting power within as little as 11 days after beginning a low-fat diet and exercise regimen.[10]

The Bottom Line

While more research will be of great value, evidence already suggests that men with prostate cancer—and their families—should be encouraged to adopt a low-fat, vegan diet. By boosting vegetables, fruits, beans, and whole grains, and avoiding dairy products, meats, eggs, and fried foods, men are able to take advantage of protective nutrients and avoid cancer-promoting factors.

Foods and Prostate Cancer References

1. Breslow N, Chan CW, Dhom G, et al. Latent carcinoma of prostate at autopsy in seven areas. Int J Cancer 1977;20:680-8.

2. Fradet Y, Meyer F, Bairati I, Shadmani R. Dietary fat and prostate cancer progression and survival. Eur Urol 1999;388:91.

3. Kim DJ, Gallagher RP, Hislop TG, et al. Premorbid diet in relation to survival from prostate cancer (Canada). Cancer Causes and Control 2000;11:65-77.

4. Ornish D, Weidner G, Fair WR, et al. Intensive lifestyle changes may affect the progression of prostate cancer. J Urol. 2005 Sep;174(3):1065-1070.

5. Carter JP, Saxe GP, Newbold V, Peres CE, Campeau RJ, Bernal-Green L. Hypothesis: Dietary management may improve survival from nutritionally linked cancers based on analysis of representative cases. J Am Coll Nutr 1993;12:209-26.

6. Saxe GA, Hebert JR, Carmody JF, et al. Can diet in conjunction with stress reduction affect the rate of increase in prostate specific antigen after biochemical recurrence of prostate cancer? J Urol 2001;266:2202-7.

7. Lee CT, Fair WR. The role of dietary manipulation in biochemical recurrence of prostate cancer after radical prostatectomy. Semin Urol 1999;17:154-63.

8. Yip I, Heber D, Aronson W. Nutrition and prostate cancer. Urol Clin N America 1999;26:403-11.

9. Tymchuk CN, Barnard RJ, Ngo TH, Aronson WJ. Role of testosterone, estradiol, and insulin in diet- and exercise-induced reductions in serum-stimulated prostate cancer cell growth in vitro. Nutr Cancer 2002;42:112-6.

10. Tymchuk CN, Barnard RJ, Heber D, Aronson WJ. Evidence of an inhibitory effect of diet and exercise on prostate cancer cell growth. J Urol 2001;166:1185-9.

Questions and Answers About Foods and Cancer Prevention and Survival

*How do you get enough **protein** on a vegan diet?*

Protein is an important nutrient required for the building, maintenance, and repair of tissues in the body. Amino acids, the building blocks of protein, can be synthesized by the body or ingested from food. There are 20 different amino acids in the food we eat, but our body can only make 11 of them. The 9 essential amino acids cannot be produced by the body and must be obtained from the diet. A variety of grains, legumes, and vegetables easily provides all of the essential amino acids our bodies require. It was once thought that various plant foods had to be eaten together to get their full protein value ("protein combining" or "protein complementing"). We now know that intentional combining is not necessary to obtain all of the essential amino acids. As long as the diet contains a variety of grains, legumes, and vegetables, protein needs are easily met.

With the traditional Western diet, the average American consumes about double the protein her or his body needs. Additionally, the main sources of protein consumed tend to be animal products, which are also high in fat and saturated fat. Most individuals are surprised to learn that their protein needs are actually much lower than what they have been consuming. The Recommended Dietary Allowance (RDA) for protein for the average, sedentary adult is only 0.8 grams per kilogram of body weight.

To find out your average individual need, simply perform the following calculation:

body weight in pounds $\times$ 0.36 = recommended protein intake in grams

However, even this value has a large margin of safety, and the body's true need is even lower for most people. Protein needs are increased for women who are pregnant or breastfeeding. In addition, needs are also higher for very active persons. As these groups require additional calories, increased protein needs can easily be met through larger intake of food consumed daily. Extra serving of legumes, tofu, meat substitutes, or other high protein sources can help meet needs that go beyond the current RDA.

*What about my **kids**? Is it ok for them to eat a vegan diet?*

Eating habits are set in early childhood. Choosing a vegetarian diet can give your child—and your whole family—the opportunity to learn to enjoy a variety of nutritious foods.

Children raised on fruits, vegetables, whole grains, and legumes grow up to be slimmer and healthier and live longer than their meat-eating friends. It is, in fact, much easier to build a nutritious diet from plant foods than from animal products, which contain saturated fat, cholesterol, and other substances that growing children can do without. As for essential nutrients, plant foods are the preferred source because they provide sufficient energy and protein packaged with health-promoting fiber, antioxidant vitamins, minerals, and phytochemicals.

Naturally, children need protein to grow, but they do not need high-protein, animal-based foods. Many people are unaware that a varied menu of grains, beans, vegetables, and fruits supplies plenty of protein. The "protein deficiencies" that our parents worried about in impoverished countries were the result of starvation or diets restricted to very few food items. Protein deficiency is extremely unlikely on a diet drawn from a variety of plant foods.

Very young children may need a slightly higher fat intake than adults do. Healthier fat sources include soybean products, avocados, and nut butters. Soy "hot dogs," peanut butter and jelly sandwiches, seasoned veggie burgers, and avocado chunks in salads, for example, are very well accepted. However, the need for fat in the diet should not be taken too far. American children often have fatty streaks in the arteries—the beginnings of heart disease—before they finish high school. In contrast, Japanese children traditionally grow up on diets much lower in fat and subsequently have fewer problems with diabetes, heart disease, obesity, and other chronic diseases.

Parents will want to make sure their child's diet includes a regular source of vitamin B_{12}, which is needed for healthy blood and nerve function. Deficiencies are rare, but when they happen, they can be a bit hard to detect. Vitamin B_{12} is plentiful in many commercial cereals, fortified soy- and rice milks, and nutritional yeast. Check the labels for the words cyanocobalamin or B_{12}. Children who do not eat these supplemented products should take a B_{12} supplement of 3 or more micrograms per day. Common children's vitamins contain more than enough B_{12}. Spirulina and seaweed are not reliable sources of vitamin B_{12}.

The body also requires vitamin D, which is normally produced by sun on the skin. Fifteen to twenty minutes of daily sunlight on the hands and face is enough for the body's skin cells to produce the necessary vitamin D. Children in latitudes with diminished sunlight may need the vitamin D found in multivitamin supplements or fortified non-dairy milks.

Good calcium sources include beans, dried figs, sweet potatoes, and green vegetables, including collards, kale, broccoli, mustard greens, and Swiss chard. Fortified soymilk and rice milk and calcium-fortified juices provide a great deal of calcium as well. In addition, eating lots of fruits and vegetables, excluding animal proteins, and limiting salt intake all help the body retain calcium.

Growing children also need iron found in a variety of beans and green leafy vegetables. The vitamin C in vegetables and fruits enhances iron absorption, especially when eaten together with an iron-rich food. One example is an iron-rich bean burrito eaten with vitamin C-rich tomato salsa. Few people are aware that cow's milk is very low in iron and can induce a mild, chronic blood loss in the digestive tract, which can reduce iron and cause an increased risk of anemia.

What is the difference between **soluble** and **insoluble fiber**?

Both soluble and insoluble fiber are valuable in preventing disease. Soluble fiber makes up about one-quarter of the fiber in food. It dissolves in water, slows digestion by slowing down the time it takes for the stomach to empty, and helps the body absorb nutrients from food. Oats, beans and other legumes, and some fruits and vegetables are all good sources of soluble fiber. Psyllium, a grain found in some cereals and in certain bulk fiber supplements, is also a good source of soluble fiber. Soluble fiber can help lower blood cholesterol, particularly if you have elevated cholesterol levels, and may help control blood sugar levels in people with diabetes.

Insoluble fiber makes up about three-quarters of the fiber in food. It does not dissolve in water, and "holds" water which helps to create bulk and moisture to the stool. The water-holding quality of insoluble fiber creates a feeling of fullness in the stomach and helps foods pass through the stomach and intestines. It's made up from the structural material of the cell walls of plants. It consists of cellulose, hemicellulose, and lignin. Insoluble fiber passes through the gastrointestinal tract mostly undigested (the human body does not have the enzymes to break down insoluble fiber). Additionally, unlike soluble fiber, insoluble fibers are *not* metabolized by intestinal bacteria. The skins of many fruits and vegetables, seeds, nuts, wheat, and whole grains (also whole-grain breads, cereals and pasta) are good sources of insoluble fiber. Though all plant cells contain both soluble and insoluble fibers in varying amounts, some foods are more abundant in one type of fiber. Some foods especially rich in the insoluble type of fiber are grapes, prunes, apple skins, pear skins, berries, celery, beets, carrots, Brussels sprouts, turnips, cabbage, cauliflower, broccoli, rhubarb, red chard, asparagus, corn, popcorn, kidney beans, potato skins, and bran.

What are the best **oils** to use in cooking? And what about **nuts**? They're healthy, right?

Although vegetable oils and nuts generally contain less saturated fatty acids than animal fats, when it comes to hormone production and the functioning of your immune system, total fat is what matters—regardless of whether or not it's a "good" or "bad" fat. For cancer prevention and survival, it's best to avoid sources of concentrated fat. Use fat-free substitutes for vegetable oils, such as vegetable broth or water, whenever possible. Nuts and nut butters should be used as a condiment at most. If oils are absolutely necessary, choose ones that are rich in omega-3 fatty acids, such as canola or walnut oil. If you eat nuts, be conscious of your serving size (it's easy to overdo it—shoot for a serving of no more than 1 tablespoon chopped nuts per day, which contains about 5 grams of fat and 50 calories), and choose nuts that are rich in essential nutrients. For example, one Brazil nut supplies you with your daily requirement of the antioxidant selenium. Almonds are good sources of calcium and vitamin E. And walnuts are rich in omega-3 fatty acids.

*I've heard that **macrobiotic diets** are great for cancer prevention and survival. What are macrobiotic diets, and what do you think of them?*

Numerous epidemiological studies have shown that a low-fat, plant-based diet based on whole grains, legumes, vegetables, and fruit is the healthiest for cancer prevention and preventing recurrence. Macrobiotics includes a number of healthful lifestyle, diet, and eating environment recommendations.

The macrobiotic diet in itself is nearly vegan. However, some people following macrobiotic diets occasionally consume fish. We discourage the consumption of fish and shellfish because their flesh contains toxic chemicals at concentrations as high as 9 million times those found in the polluted water in which they swim. Mercury, found in especially high levels in tuna and swordfish, can cause brain damage. This is of particular concern to growing children. Pesticides, such as DDT, PCBs, and dioxin, have been linked to cancers, nervous system disorders, fetal damage, and many other health problems. Avoiding fish eliminates half of all mercury exposure and reduces one's intake of other toxins as well, not to mention the fact that fish flesh provides excessive amounts of protein, fat, and cholesterol, with no cancer-fighting fiber, complex carbohydrates, or vitamin C. Many people say they eat fish rather than beef in hopes of limiting fat and cholesterol. But many fish, such as catfish, swordfish, and sea trout, contain almost one-third fat. Salmon is 52 percent fat. And, ounce for ounce, shrimp have double the cholesterol of beef.

*I've heard that you need to get certain **essential oils** in your diet and that fish are a good source. Are there plant sources of these essential oils?*

Two essential fatty acids cannot be synthesized in the body and must be taken in the diet from plant foods. Their names—linoleic and linolenic acid—will never show up on a food label and are not important to remember. What *is* important is that these basic fats are used to build specialized fats called omega-3 and omega-6 fatty acids.

Omega-3 and omega-6 fatty acids are important in the normal functioning of all tissues of the body. Deficiencies are responsible for a host of symptoms and disorders including abnormalities in the liver and kidneys, changes in the blood, reduced growth rates, decreased immune function, and skin changes including dryness and scaliness. Adequate intake of the essential fatty acids results in numerous health benefits. Prevention of atherosclerosis, reduced incidence of heart disease and stroke, and relief from the symptoms associated with ulcerative colitis, menstrual pain, and joint pain have also been documented.

While supplements and added oils are not typically necessary, good sources of omega-3 fats should be part of a daily diet. Alpha-linoleic acid (ALA), a common omega-3 fatty acid, is found in many vegetables, beans, and fruits. More concentrated sources can be found in oils such as canola, flaxseed, soybean, walnut, and wheat germ. Corn, safflower, sunflower, and cottonseed oils are generally low in ALA. Omega-6 fatty acids, such as gamma-linolenic acid, can be found in more rare oils, including black currant, borage, evening primrose, and hemp oils.

Some people eat fish and use fish oils for their omega-3s. However, plant-derived omegas-3s have none of the fish odor that can be apparent in the perspiration of people using fish oil. They also tend to be more chemically stable and are lower in saturated fats. Fish oils tend to decompose and unleash dangerous free radicals in the process. Another downside to fish oils is that they are between 15 and 30 percent saturated fat, which is about double that of plant oils. Fish oils are in no way unique. Fish make their omega-3 oils from ALA in plankton, just as mammals—including humans—synthesize omega-3s from land plants. Research has shown that omega-3s are found in a more stable form in vegetables, fruits, and beans. Adding flaxseed oil to your salad or grinding flax seeds for your breakfast cereal are simple ways to incorporate extra omega-3 fatty acids to your diet.

*Other than the essential fatty acids in **flaxseeds**, isn't there another reason **why breast cancer survivors** should eat them?*

A recent Canadian study examined the effect of consuming flaxseed oil on tumor growth in postmenopausal women with breast cancer. Twenty-nine women were assigned to either eat a muffin containing 25 grams of flaxseed oil or a muffin with no flaxseed oil. The flaxseed oil muffins offered some clear benefits, as the majority of the women eating them had a significant reduction in breast cell tumor size. This effect is similar to that seen with tamoxifen, a drug given to some women to prevent breast cancer. The drug acts as a selective estrogen receptor modifier (SERM), and flaxseed, which is rich in plant-based estrogens, appears to act in a similar way.

Want to incorporate more flaxseed into your diet? Try adding ground flaxseed to salads, soups, casseroles, and cereals. You can also top salads with flaxseed oil. Store ground flaxseeds and flaxseed oil in your refrigerator to keep them fresh and to avoid rancidity. The best way to use flaxseed is as an addition to a low-fat, vegan diet.

*I've read that **milk consumption decreases risk for breast cancer** in premenopausal women. How could this be if milk consumption increases a woman's level of IGF-I and may increase breast cancer risk after menopause?*

A study in Norway in 2001 created a stir, because it concluded that milk consumption reduces breast cancer risk in premenopausal women. But, breast cancer is quite uncommon in premenopausal women (only 0.6 percent in this study). Also, the study relied solely on self-reported milk intake during adulthood and the *recollection* of milk intake during childhood, not on key blood markers related to breast cancer risk or overall dairy product intake.

The nutrient that is hypothesized to be protective is conjugated linoleic acid (CLA), a component of dairy fat, which has been shown to increase risk for heart disease. A number of other studies have shown either no association between breast cancer incidence and dairy product consumption or an *increase* between the two. Research has shown that foods influence breast cancer development by their actions on circulating hormone levels (especially estrogen). Fatty foods increase estrogen levels while high-fiber foods naturally decrease them. High-fat diets also fuel obesity, which is associated with elevated estrogen and increased breast cancer risk.

In Asia, where whole grains, vegetables, fruits, tofu, soymilk, and other soy products are commonly consumed and milk is not a normal part of the diet, people are generally healthier and breast cancer is much rarer than in the United States and Europe.

*Aside from not smoking, are there any **lifestyle factors** that help decrease risk for **lung cancer**?*

A study published in *Lancet* in 2000 suggests that the natural chemicals in broccoli, cabbage, bok choy, and other cruciferous vegetables may protect against lung cancer. Of 18,000 men studied, those with detectable *isothiocyanate*, a phytochemical, in their blood had a 36 percent lower chance of developing lung cancer than those with none.

Researchers warned the public not to depend on vegetables as infallible immunity against the strong cancer-causing effects of smoking or to rely on isothiocyanate supplements if they are ever produced. More than 20 different varieties of these compounds work intricately together in the body in ways that can't be duplicated in pill form. In fact, antioxidants taken in doses higher than those which occur naturally in plant foods can actually increase cancer risk. The lesson, report investigators, is simple: "Just eat your vegetables, and lots of them."

*I'm having trouble **keeping weight on**. What are some healthy plant-based snacks that will help me keep weight on?*

Dry beans and peas, nuts, peanut butter, and seeds are examples of foods commonly eaten by non-vegetarians, but perhaps not very often or in small quantities. These can supply a greater percentage of calorie and protein requirements. Shakes can be made with soymilk, tofu, and non-dairy frozen desserts and can be flavored with fruit, chocolate syrup, or extracts to make a tasty, calorie-rich treat. Also, many varieties of trail mix are readily available and great for high-energy snacking.

*Can a plant-based diet reduce the risk of **testicular cancer**?*

There isn't a wealth of literature showing that a plant-based diet or any particular diet decreases a man's risk for developing testicular cancer. However, some evidence links dairy products, such as cheese, to testicular cancer, just as dairy products appear to be linked to prostate cancer. Fatty foods generally escalate testosterone activity, which may mean higher cancer risk over the long run. There are also other biological mechanisms linking fatty foods and cancer risk.

*How important is it to eat **organic food** (e.g., to avoid pesticides and other carcinogens)?*

Buying organic produce is a good idea, particularly for strawberries, bell peppers, spinach, cherries, and peaches—the produce items containing the highest concentration of pesticide residues, according to data from the U.S. Food and Drug Administration.

Another great way to avoid concentrated sources of pesticides is to avoid meat because pesticides on cattle feed become concentrated in the tissues of the animals.

*What about **soy products**? Are the **phytoestrogens** in soy foods helpful or risky for cancer survivors? Do estrogens in soy increase breast cancer risk? What about the estrogens in soy for men and boys?*

Soy products, such as miso soup, tofu, and tempeh, contain very weak plant estrogens called *phytoestrogens* that hinder the body's natural estrogen from attaching to cells. (The prefix "phyto" simply means "plant.") Normally, estrogens hook onto tiny receptor proteins in your cells that allow them to change the cell's chemistry.

Think of it this way: An estrogen molecule is like a jumbo jet that attaches to the Jetway of an airport. It discharges passengers into the terminal, which is suddenly a busy, noisy place. Phytoestrogens, being weak estrogens, are like small, private planes with few passengers and no cargo, yet they still occupy the Jetway after landing. When phytoestrogens occupy the cell, normal estrogens cannot. Plant estrogens do not eliminate all of estrogen's effects, but they do minimize them, apparently reducing breast cancer risk and menstrual symptoms.

For men and boys, the phytoestrogens in soy do not appear to have any effect on hormone levels and have not been shown to affect sexual development or fertility. Research studies show that men consuming soy have less prostate cancer and better prostate cancer survival.

In Asia, where tofu, soymilk, and other soy products are commonly consumed, not only is the population healthier overall, but cancer and heart disease are much rarer than in the United States and Europe, and longevity is greater. As these populations differ in other ways—Asians eat much less meat and dairy products and generally exercise more, but they also smoke more cigarettes and eat more salt—researchers have simply attempted to tease out the effects of soy itself. Also, it's possible that the more processed soy products, such as veggie burgers and veggie hot dogs, are not as beneficial as the less processed soy products, such as tofu and tempeh, traditionally consumed in Asia. In general, the less processed your diet is, the more nutrient-dense it will be. Thus, replacing processed soy products such as veggie burgers and veggie hot dogs with tofu, tempeh, beans, and lentils may provide you with a more nutrient-dense diet.

Research findings are not clear on whether soy products are safe for women who have had breast cancer. Some researchers believe that two servings per day of soy products such as soymilk, tofu, or tempeh are fine for these women, and others discourage soy consumption completely. If your oncologist or physician has told you to avoid soy, it's important to listen to those recommendations.

Like all foods, soy has its advantages and disadvantages. Soybeans are rich in essential omega-3 fatty acids but tend to be higher in total fat than other beans. Many soy products derive roughly half their calories from fat, while black beans, pinto beans, or other varieties are only about 4 percent fat. Also, soy extracts, such as genistein, may not have the same beneficial effects as products made with the whole bean.

However, it's also to remember that a vegan diet of beans, vegetables, grains, and fruits does not have to include soy products to be nutritionally complete. Soy products make convenient and tasty substitutes for meat and other unhealthy foods that people, quite rightly, are looking to avoid. However, the benefits of complete protein and soluble fiber can easily be found in an array of plant foods.

In human research studies, soy products have been shown to lower serum cholesterol levels, in part due to their rich content of soluble fiber, and the isoflavones also play a role in bone formation. Soy products have been shown to reduce estrogen activity, at least in premenopausal women, which, over the long run, reduces cancer risk. The evidence is not as clear for postmenopausal women.

What about **raw vegan diets**? Are they even better than vegan diets that include cooked foods?

The Cancer Project has not yet evaluated the research on the health benefits of raw food diets. However, a low-fat diet that is rich in raw or cooked vegetables, fruits, and other plant-based foods is loaded with antioxidants and other cancer-fighting nutrients and has been shown in numerous studies to have the most disease-protecting power of any diet regimen. There are significant advantages to having vegetables and fruits in their raw form since cooking sometimes causes the loss of some nutrients that are powerful antioxidants and help protect us from developing cancer. However, there are foods that become more nutrient-dense when cooked, as seen with the increased lycopene activity in cooked tomatoes, for example. Lycopene intake has been shown to reduce the risk for developing prostate cancer. Also, some foods, such as cruciferous vegetables (e.g., broccoli, Brussels sprouts) are difficult to eat raw. However, there is no doubt that humans existed on uncooked foods throughout most of our evolution, even though it is not clear which plant foods were dominant in the diet of early humans.

Does **cooking** vegetables generally destroy cancer-fighting compounds?

Water-soluble nutrients, such as vitamin C and the B vitamins, do seep out of foods during boiling or steaming. However, if you reuse the cooking liquid in soups or to cook grains, you will get all the nutrients that have seeped out of the vegetables. On the contrary, some antioxidants are actually released or activated by cooking, including the lycopene in tomatoes and the beta-carotene in carrots and sweet potatoes. Researchers have found that you can multiply the antioxidant power of your carrots three times by cooking and puréeing them before eating. It turns out that cooking and puréeing releases cancer-fighting compounds from the carrot cells. To reap the full cancer-fighting benefits from the carrots you prepare, wash them thoroughly, but avoid peeling them as the skins are rich with cancer-fighting compounds. Also, try these tips to increase the beta-carotene in your diet:
- When making mashed potatoes, add 2 carrots to the pot of potatoes when you boil them. Then mash the two vegetables together for a delicious and conversation-starting result.
- Try making a carrot soup with 6 carrots boiled in just enough water

to cover them. When the carrots are soft, purée them with the cooking liquid in a blender or food processor. Add 1 cup of orange juice and 1 teaspoon of grated ginger and salt and pepper to taste. Heat and serve.

Do you recommend taking the popular "green food" **supplements** *that are on the market now? Will they help prevent cancer?*

Vegetable-based supplements are increasing in popularity and often come with a variety of health claims. It is important to consider, however, that no single supplement can replicate all the healthy components found in a variety of whole plant foods, including those that ward off cancer.

Vegetables, fruits, whole grains, and legumes are packed with lots of healthful substances *beyond* vitamins, such as fiber, minerals, and cancer-protective phytochemicals. Increasing your fruits and veggies can be almost as simple as popping a pill and is far more beneficial.

Try these simple ideas to get your five (and more) servings a day:
- Add vitamin-rich veggies, like bell peppers, broccoli, carrots, tomatoes, and spinach, to salads.
- Add cooked, puréed pumpkin to soups and stews as a thickener.
- Take a bowl of fruit to work each week (apples, bananas, pears, oranges) and snack from it throughout the day.
- Pack raisins and other dried fruits in your purse, briefcase, or backpack to keep you fueled with healthy foods.

One supplement that is important, however, is vitamin B_{12}, which is needed for healthy blood and healthy nerves. It is found in any common multiple vitamin, as well as in simple B_{12} supplements. It is also found in fortified cereals (e.g., Product 19, Total, Kellogg's Corn Flakes), fortified soymilks, and some brands of nutritional yeast.

How do fruit and vegetable **juices** *compare to eating them whole?*

One-half a cup (4 ounces) of juice can be considered the equivalent of a single serving of fruits or vegetables. As a rule of thumb, it's important to shoot for consuming at least 3 servings of fruit and 3 servings of vegetables every day. However, since juice is not as high in fiber as whole fruit or vegetables, it's always best to consume the whole food whenever possible. It has been shown that diets higher in fiber are not only beneficial for protecting against a number of cancers and chronic illnesses, but also help you fill up so that you don't "fill out"—and maintaining a healthy weight is yet another way to ward off cancer.

Juicing fruits and vegetables can be a great way for people who don't enjoy eating lots of fruits and vegetables to bring these healthy plant foods into their routine—and the juicers that keep the fiber in the foods are best. Or, the fibrous end-product that juicers produce can be re-used (instead of discarded): shredded carrots make a salad topping, for example, or they can be thrown into soups, stir-fries, or pasta sauces.

*If a **completely plant-based diet isn't possible** for me, is it ok if I can at least eliminate red meat and cheese and eat a low-fat diet with egg whites, chicken, fish, and skim milk in addition to lots of fruits and vegetables?*

A low-fat, completely vegan diet is the healthiest diet of all. It's naturally high in fiber and cholesterol-free—two proven means to reduce cancer risk. Eliminating red meat and cheese is a start. However, you'll want to go one step further, and base your diet on whole grains, legumes, vegetables, and fruit. You'll get much higher doses of cancer fighting vitamins, minerals, fiber, and phytochemicals. Although skim milk and egg whites are lower in fat than whole milk and whole eggs, these foods—as well as chicken and fish—contain high amounts of cholesterol and other harmful compounds, so they should be avoided completely. An easy way to shift to a completely plant-based diet is to do it 100 percent for three solid weeks. It will take your body that amount of time to adjust to new flavors and tastes and get used to not having some of the foods you've been eating all your life. Those 21 days will fly by. When you reach the end of three weeks, evaluate how you feel—you'll realize that you feel a lot better and lighter and that you don't miss the high-fat foods you had been used to.

*For an **overweight** breast cancer survivor, is it important to just focus on eating healthy, or is weight loss important too?*

You'll want to focus on both. Evidence suggests you can improve your chances of surviving breast cancer and reduce recurrence by achieving a healthy weight post-treatment. The best way to lose weight is to choose healthy, low-fat meals built from legumes, grains, vegetables, and fruit, and to incorporate moderate physical activity into your lifestyle. Of course, it's important to check with your doctor to get the green light for the type and level of exercise you'd like to do. You'll feel better for it!

*What vitamins and minerals are important to take to protect someone with a history of **prostate cancer**? What foods are best?*

In addition to avoiding dairy products and emphasizing lycopene-rich foods, such as tomatoes, watermelon, or pink grapefruit in your diet, there may be value in paying attention to the mineral selenium.

When researchers compared blood samples of men with prostate cancer to age-similar controls without cancer, they found that men with prostate cancer had lower levels of serum selenium. Another study hypothesized that this protective effect of selenium may be due to the mineral's ability to raise plasma levels of 25-hydroxyvitamin D, the active form of vitamin D.

So, how can you protect yourself against prostate cancer? Whole grains are a good source of selenium, so get started by choosing a vegan diet rich in whole grains. Replace dairy products with vegetable sources of calcium, such as leafy greens and legumes. And add some tomatoes to your salad.

How important is diet for young girls in families with a **history of breast cancer**?

The foods girls eat while in pre-school and grade school appear to have an important effect on breast cancer risk later in life. Researchers at Harvard have discovered that girls who eat more protein from animal sources and less protein from plant sources tended to reach menarche earlier. Younger age at first menstruation is connected with increased risk of breast cancer later in life.

Do you have to eat **garlic** raw to get its health benefits?

Cook onions and garlic in an open skillet and nearly anyone who walks into your house will tell you how good it smells. The same sulfur-containing substances that make onions and garlic so aromatic are excellent cancer fighters. The protective chemicals in garlic and onions appear to block carcinogens from reaching their targets, destroy cancer cells, and suppress tumor growth.

Eaten regularly, garlic and onions are associated with as much as a 50 to 60 percent decreased risk of stomach and colorectal cancers. The cancer fighters in these tasty foods work whether they are raw or cooked, so enjoy fresh onions sliced on your veggie burger or as a topping for your black bean soup, or roast whole heads of garlic in the oven and spread the cloves (naturally softened and sweetened by cooking) onto bread or crackers to take advantage of the benefits of these foods.

Cooking temperatures can eliminate garlic's beneficial effects on cells unless the garlic is allowed to stand for about 10 minutes between being crushed and the cooking process.

How do **dairy** products cause cancer? And if you don't drink milk, how do you get all the **calcium** you need?

Recent scientific studies have suggested that specific components in dairy products may be linked to an increased risk for ovarian, breast, and prostate cancers. For ovarian cancer, galactose, a component of the milk sugar lactose, has been under study as a possible culprit. In prostate cancer, both the fat content and the high calcium content may play a role. In addition, dairy product consumption has been shown to increase levels of insulin-like growth factor I (IGF-I) in the body, a potent stimulus for cancer cell growth. High IGF-I levels are linked to increased risk of prostate cancer and breast cancer.

Replace cow's milk in your diet with healthier alternatives, such as rice milk, almond milk, and soymilk. If you're having trouble giving up ice cream, try Rice Dream and Tofutti brand frozen desserts. There are even a number of cheese, cream cheese, sour cream, and yogurt alternatives readily available in grocery and health food stores. As you eliminate dairy products from your diet, you may notice that your body is also benefiting in other ways with an improvement in digestion, a reduction in arthritis pain, and fewer symptoms of seasonal and/or other allergies.

What about calcium? There's plenty of easily absorbed calcium in dark leafy greens, such as bok choy, kale, mustard greens, collard greens, and turnip greens, as well as broccoli, dried beans, soy nuts, figs, almonds, calcium-fortified juices, and soymilk and other non-dairy milks. Plus, these foods contain other cancer-fighting nutrients that aren't present in dairy products.

How Much Calcium Is Absorbed from Foods?

For comparison, 32% of the calcium from dairy products is absorbed.

Food Source	Calcium Absorption Percentage Rate
Beans, white	17.0 %
Broccoli	52.6 %
Brussels sprouts	63.8 %
Kale	58.8 %
Kohlrabi	67.0 %
Mustard greens	57.8 %
Orange juice, calcium fortified	37.0 %
Soymilk	31.0 %
Tofu, calcium set	31.0 %
Turnip greens	51.6 %

*How do you ensure proper **food safety** when cooking for someone undergoing chemotherapy?*

A clean and safe food supply is healthy for everyone, but it is especially important for people with compromised immune systems. Older persons and individuals undergoing cancer treatment can be especially at risk from bacteria, viruses, or other foreign substances that can turn up in food. To keep your meals safe and clean, follow these simple practices:

- Wash hands with soapy water before and after preparing food and before eating.
- Avoid preparing or eating all types of meat, eggs, and dairy products, as these foods are most likely to be contaminated with bacteria. Poultry products are especially likely to be contaminated. Raw milk and home-prepared ice creams or mayonnaise, as well as cake and cookie batter made with eggs, may easily contain infectious bacteria.

- Keep cold foods cold (below 40°F) and hot foods hot (above 165°F).
- Wash fruits and vegetables thoroughly under running water before using them.
- Wash the tops of cans before opening.
- During food preparation, if you taste the food you are making, use a different utensil than the one used for stirring or serving.
- Do not taste food that looks or smells strange.

Recipes

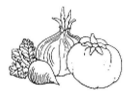

Table of Contents

Appetizers

Cheesy Garbanzo Spread

Makes about 2 cups

This delicious spread has the look and taste of spreadable cheese and takes only seconds to prepare. Try it on bread and crackers, in casseroles, and as a filling for quesadillas. Look for jars of water-packed roasted red peppers near the pickles and olives in your supermarket. Tahini is available in the ethnic food section of many supermarkets and in natural food stores.

1 15-ounce can garbanzo beans
1/2 cup roasted red peppers
3 tablespoons tahini (sesame seed butter)
3 tablespoons lemon juice

Drain the garbanzo beans, reserving the liquid, and set the liquid aside. Place the beans in a food processor or blender with the roasted red peppers, tahini, and lemon juice. Process until very smooth. If using a blender, you will have to stop it occasionally and push everything down into the blades with a rubber spatula. The mixture should be quite thick, but if it is too thick to blend, add a tablespoon or two of the reserved bean liquid.

Recipe from Eat Right, Live Longer *by Neal D. Barnard, M.D.;*
recipe by Jennifer Raymond

Creamy Spinach Dip

Serves 10 to 12

Great for a family gathering or as a dish to pass for a holiday cocktail party.

1 container non-dairy (vegan) sour cream substitute, or 1 container (8 oz.)
   vegan cream cheese plus 1/4 cup water
1 tablespoon lemon juice
1/2 cup salsa
1 package frozen chopped spinach, thawed and drained
1 package vegetable soup mix

Combine ingredients and refrigerate for 1 hour before serving. Serve with raw vegetable pieces or chunks of crusty bread.

Recipe adapted from old family favorite by PCRM
nutrition director Amy Lanou, Ph.D.

Guacamole Plus

Makes 2 1/2 cups

This guacamole is enriched with fiber from the peas and cancer-fighting phytochemicals from the garlic, salsa, scallions, and lemon.

1 cup frozen green peas or 1 cup drained and rinsed canned peas
1 ripe avocado, peeled
1/2 cup mild salsa
1 clove garlic, minced, or 1 teaspoon chopped garlic
1 scallion, minced *(optional)*
juice of 1 lemon
1/2 teaspoon cumin
1 tablespoon fresh cilantro, chopped *(optional)*
salt and pepper, to taste

If using frozen peas, blanch peas in boiling water for 2 minutes, then cool with cold water and drain. Cut avocado into large chunks. Mash avocado and peas together using a potato masher or fork, or, if a very creamy texture is desired, in a food processor. Mix in salsa, garlic, scallion (if using), lemon juice, cumin, and cilantro (if using). Add salt and pepper to taste.

Hummus

Makes about 2 cups

1 can garbanzo beans
2 tablespoons tahini (sesame butter)
1/4 cup lemon juice
3 scallions, chopped
1 tablespoon chopped garlic (about 3 cloves)
1 teaspoon cumin
1/2 teaspoon black pepper
1/2 cup roasted red peppers *(optional)*

Drain garbanzo beans, reserving the liquid from the can, and rinse the beans.

Place all ingredients except reserved bean liquid in food processor and process until smooth. Add reserved bean liquid as needed for a smoother consistency.

Spread on whole-wheat pita bread or serve as a dip for vegetables.

Recipe by PCRM dietitian Jennifer Keller, R.D.

Mockamole

Serves 6

If you long for your favorite south-of-the-border dip but don't want the fat of avocado, try this reduced-fat version of guacamole. You can use either green peas or green beans for part of the avocado. Green peas will give this dip a slightly sweet flavor that we found especially appealing.

1 avocado
2 cups cooked peas or 1 cup cooked green beans
2 tablespoons chopped onion
1/4 cup salsa (or more to taste)
2 tablespoons fresh lime juice
salt to taste

Blend the avocado and peas or green beans together in a blender, until smooth. Stir in the onion and salsa. Just before serving, stir in the fresh lime juice and salt. Serve with baked tortilla chips.

Recipe from The Vegetarian No-Cholesterol Family-Style Cookbook *by Kate Schumann and Virginia Messina, M.P.H., R.D.*

Roasted Sweet Potato Wedges

Serves 4

2 medium-sized sweet potatoes, cut into wedges
1/8 teaspoon cinnamon
1/4 teaspoon season salt
1/4 teaspoon ground cumin
1/8 teaspoon pepper
1/4 teaspoon garlic powder

Preheat oven to 450°F.

Combine all ingredients in a plastic bag. Seal and shake. Place sweet potato wedges on a baking sheet coated with cooking spray (do not overlap). Bake at 450°F for 20 minutes or until very tender, flipping potatoes once during cooking.

Recipe from PCRM Weight Loss Study Cooking Demonstration; contributed by PCRM dietitian Brie Turner-McGrievy, M.S., R.D.

Tomato Corn Salsa

Makes 3 1/2 cups

Corn adds fiber and color to this lycopene-rich dip or topping.

1 cup fresh or frozen corn kernels, thawed
2 cups diced tomatoes
2 tablespoons diced red onions
1/4 cup diced green bell peppers
1 tablespoon chopped fresh basil
1/2 to 1 fresh green chile, minced or 1/2 to 1 teaspoon of your favorite
   chili sauce
1 tablespoon fresh lime juice
1 teaspoon rice or cider vinegar

If corn is not thawed completely, either blanch it in boiling water to cover
for 1 to 2 minutes, or microwave it until thawed. Drain. In a large bowl,
combine all of the ingredients and set aside for 15 to 20 minutes to allow
the flavors to develop. Add salt, if desired and serve at room temperature.

Recipe adapted from Moosewood Restaurant Low-Fat Favorites
by The Moosewood Collective

Veggies in a Blanket

Makes 40 individual pieces

8 flour tortillas
1/2 cup non-dairy (vegan) cream cheese substitute or hummus
4 grated carrots
8 lettuce leaves, a couple handfuls of baby spinach leaves, or 1 container
   sprouts

Warm tortillas in a dry pan, if desired. Spread vegan cream cheese or hummus on the tortillas. Add carrots and lettuce, spinach, or sprouts. Roll up
each tortilla, secure each with 5 evenly placed toothpicks, and slice into 5
individual rolls per tortilla (one toothpick per roll).

Variations: Add thin sticks of cucumber or sweet red pepper before rolling.

Soups, Chowders, Chilis, and Stews

Carrot and Red Pepper Soup
Serves 4

1 onion, chopped
6 carrots, thinly sliced
2 cups water or vegetable stock
2 red bell peppers
2 cups soymilk
2 teaspoons lemon juice
2 teaspoons balsamic vinegar
1/2 teaspoon salt
1/4 teaspoon freshly ground black pepper

Place the onion and carrots in a pot with the water, and simmer, covered, over medium heat until the carrots can be easily pierced with a fork, about 20 minutes.

Meanwhile, roast the peppers by placing them over an open gas flame or directly under the broiler until the skin is completely blackened. Place in a bowl, cover, and let stand about 15 minutes. Slip the charred skin off with your fingers, then cut the peppers in half and remove the seeds.

Blend the carrot mixture along with the peppers in several small batches. Add some of the soymilk to each batch to facilitate blending. Return to the pot and add the lemon juice, vinegar, salt, and pepper. Heat until steamy.

Recipe from Eat Right, Live Longer *by Neal D. Barnard, M.D.;*
recipe by Jennifer Raymond

Carrot Soup

This recipe comes from Geoff Bailey at a bowling club not far from Sydney Harbor.

1 tablespoon olive oil
2 pounds (about 5 cups) peeled and sliced carrots
1 onion, chopped
2 medium potatoes, peeled and diced
6 cups water
(continued on next page)

(Carrot Soup continued)

2 cups vegetable stock
1/2 teaspoon salt
1 teaspoon sugar
black pepper to taste
1 teaspoon mixed herbs
parsley to garnish

Heat oil in a large saucepan. Add vegetables and cook over medium heat, turning with a wooden spoon until the vegetables are thoroughly coated with oil. Add water, stock, salt, sugar, pepper, and herbs. Simmer until tender. Pour into a blender and blend until smooth.

Serve with parsley.

Recipe from The Neutral Bay Club, North Sydney, Australia, printed in The Best in the World, *edited by Neal D. Barnard, M.D.*

Corn Chowder
Serves 5

1 tablespoon oil
1 onion, chopped
2 cups water
2 stalks celery, chopped
2 carrots, chopped
2 17-ounce cans vegan creamed corn
1 cup soymilk
1 potato, chopped
1 1/2 teaspoons garlic powder
1/4 teaspoon nutmeg
salt and pepper to taste

Sauté onion in oil over medium-high heat until soft. Add water, celery, and carrots. Cook 10 minutes. Add creamed corn, soymilk, potato, and spices. Continue cooking for another 10 minutes. Serve hot.

Recipe from Simply Vegan *by Debra Wasserman*

Creamy Beet Soup
Makes about 3 cups

This soup is delicious hot or cold.

1 15-ounce can diced beets
1 cup fortified soymilk or rice milk
2 tablespoons apple juice concentrate
1 teaspoon balsamic vinegar
1/2 teaspoon dried dill weed

(continued on next page)

(Creamy Beet Soup continued)

Place diced beets, including liquid, into a blender. Add soy- or rice milk, apple juice concentrate, vinegar, and dill weed. Blend on high speed until completely smooth, 2 to 3 minutes.

Transfer to a medium saucepan and heat gently until steamy.

Recipe from Healthy Eating for Life for Cancer
by Vesanto Melina, M.S., R.D.

Curried Sweet Potato Soup

Serves 6

2 teaspoons olive oil
1 cup chopped onion
2 teaspoons curry powder
1 cup water
4 cups vegetable broth
5 cups peeled, cubed sweet potato
1 1/2 cups plain soy yogurt, divided
minced cilantro *(optional)*

Heat the olive oil in a large saucepan over medium-high heat. Add the onion and curry powder and sauté for 2 minutes. Add the water, broth, and sweet potatoes. Cook for 30 minutes or until the sweet potatoes are tender. Place one-third of the sweet potato mixture in a blender and process until smooth. Repeat the procedure with the remaining sweet potato mixture in batches. Return the puréed mixture to the saucepan. Bring the soup to a boil and remove from heat. Stir in 1 cup of soy yogurt until blended. Top each serving with about 1 tablespoon of soy yogurt and garnish with cilantro, if desired.

Recipe from a PCRM Weight Loss Study Cooking Demonstration;
contributed by PCRM dietitian Brie Turner-McGrievy, M.S., R.D.

Easy Chili

Serves 4

This is a very laid-back recipe. Feel free to experiment with seasonings or try different ingredients like tofu or additional veggies.

1 large onion, chopped
1 tablespoon olive oil
2 16-ounce cans kidney beans
1 16-ounce can diced or crushed tomatoes
1 cup frozen corn
2 tablespoon chili powder
2 teaspoon cumin

(continued on next page)

(Easy Chili continued)
salt to taste
pepper to taste
garlic powder to taste

In a large skillet, sauté the onion in the olive oil. Add the beans, tomatoes, corn, and seasonings. Cover and simmer for 15 minutes to 2 hours—longer cooking time will allow the flavors to mix and yield an even tastier dish.

Kale-and-Rice Chowder

Serves 6

2 teaspoons olive oil
1 cup chopped onion
1 cup chopped red bell pepper
1/2 cup chopped leeks
1/3 cup sliced almonds
1 tablespoon paprika
2 bay leaves
1 1/2 cups water
1 14.5-ounce can seasoned, diced stewed tomatoes
2 cups vegetable broth
2 cups chopped kale
1 cup cooked brown rice
1 cup drained canned garbanzo beans

Heat the oil in a large Dutch oven over medium-high heat. Add the onion, pepper, and leeks. Sauté for 2 minutes. Add the almonds, paprika, bay leaves, water, tomatoes, and broth. Bring to a boil. Add the kale, rice, and garbanzo beans. Reduce heat and simmer 10 minutes or until thoroughly heated.

Recipe from a PCRM Weight Loss Study Cooking Demonstration; contributed by PCRM dietitian Brie Turner-McGrievy, M.S., R.D.

Lentil Artichoke Stew

Serves 4-6

This aromatic, fiber-packed, tasty Middle Eastern dish is great served over brown rice or your favorite pasta.

2 cups diced onions
2 large garlic cloves, pressed or minced
2 teaspoons ground cumin
1 teaspoon ground coriander
1 cup dry red lentils
1 bay leaf

(continued on next page)

(Lentil and Artichoke Stew continued)

1 teaspoon olive oil
2 tablespoons fresh lemon juice
2 24-ounce cans chopped tomatoes, undrained (use fire-roasted canned tomatoes if available)
1 1/2 cups quartered artichoke bottoms (9-ounce package frozen or 15-ounce can, drained)
1/4 teaspoon crushed red pepper flakes *(optional)*
water as needed
salt and ground black pepper to taste

Heat the olive oil in a saucepan. Add the onions and sauté on medium heat for about 5 minutes, until golden. Add the garlic, cumin, and coriander and cook for 2 minutes, stirring frequently. Add the lentils, bay leaf, lemon juice, tomatoes and tomato liquid, artichoke hearts, and crushed red pepper (if using), and bring to a boil. Lower the heat and simmer for about 20 minutes or until the lentils are tender. Add water if stew becomes too thick. Remove and discard the bay leaf.

Add salt and pepper to taste and serve alone or over rice or pasta.

Recipe adapted from Moosewood Restaurant Low-Fat Favorites *by The Moosewood Collective*

Lentil Soup

Serves 6

1 tablespoon olive oil
3 onions, coarsely chopped
2 cups dried lentils, rinsed
2 medium carrots, chopped
3 garlic cloves, finely chopped
1 15-ounce can of tomato sauce
2 tablespoons chopped fresh oregano
6–8 cups of water
1 large bay leaf
1/4 cup wine vinegar
1 whole potato, boiled and mashed *(optional)*
salt and freshly ground pepper to taste

In a large soup pot, add all the ingredients except for the wine vinegar and potato. Cover, bring to a boil, reduce heat to low and simmer for 1–1 1/2 hours, or until lentils are very tender. Add more water if necessary. Before removing from heat, add the wine vinegar, and, if desired, the mashed potato. Season with salt and pepper to taste.

Recipe from the Stage Door Deli Café, New York City, New York, printed in The Best in the World II, *edited by Jennifer Keller, R.D.*

Mexican Pumpkin Stew

Serves 6

Linda Arcadia of Moscow, Idaho, created this spicy soup with the rich flavors of autumn. She suggests that for a festive fall meal, you can serve this in a scooped-out pumpkin.

3–4 cups of small chunk (1/2 inch) raw pumpkin or butternut squash
1 cup vegetable stock
1 medium onion, thinly sliced
1 teaspoon minced garlic
1 cup tomato sauce
1/2 cup salsa
1 16-ounce can corn kernels, drained
1 teaspoon chili powder
1/2 teaspoon cumin
3–4 drops of Tabasco *(optional)*
1/2 teaspoon hot red pepper flakes
1 15-ounce can red kidney or pinto beans
salt and pepper to taste

Simmer the pumpkin or squash in the vegetable stock until tender. Add the remaining ingredients and simmer uncovered over low heat for 30 minutes. Season with salt and pepper.

Recipe from The Vegetarian No-Cholesterol Family-Style Cookbook
by Kate Schumann and Virginia Messina, M.P.H., R.D.

Mushroom Barley Soup

Makes about 3 cups

This soup takes just minutes to make if you have cooked barley on hand.

2 cups plain rice milk
2 tablespoons barley flour
1 cup cooked barley
1 4-ounce can mushrooms, including the liquid
1/4 teaspoon garlic powder
1/4 teaspoon salt
pinch each of dried marjoram, sage, thyme, and dill weed

Place rice milk and barley flour into a blender. Blend on high speed for a few seconds. Add barley and blend on high for about 10 seconds or until barley is chopped coarse.

Add mushrooms with their liquid. Blend just enough to coarse-chop mushrooms.

Transfer the blended mixture to a medium-sized saucepan and add all the remaining ingredients. Cook over medium heat, stirring often, for about 5

(continued on next page)

(Mushroom Barley Soup continued)

minutes, or until the soup is hot and somewhat thickened.

Recipe from Foods That Fight Pain *by Neal D. Barnard, M.D.;*
recipe by Jennifer Raymond

Posole (Vegetable Soup with Hominy)

Serves 4

Soup:
1 large onion, chopped
3 cloves garlic, minced
4 carrots, sliced
3 cups of water or low-sodium vegetable stock
1 15-ounce can of white hominy
1 15-ounce can of stewed tomatoes with garlic, green pepper, and celery
1 red pepper, chopped
1 cup green beans, broken into bite-sized lengths
1/2 teaspoon cumin
1/2 teaspoon salt, optional
1/4 teaspoon pepper
3/4 teaspoon chili powder

Toppings:
your favorite salsa
iceberg lettuce, chopped
baked tortilla chips

In a medium stockpot, braise garlic and onion in 1/2 cup of water until soft. Add carrots and water or stock, and simmer 5 to 10 minutes. Drain and rinse hominy and add to the pot. Stir in the tomatoes, red pepper, green beans, and spices. Simmer for 15 minutes. Serve piping hot with little bowls of the toppings. Add them to taste as you enjoy the soup.

Recipe from PCRM Weight Loss Study Cooking Demonstration;
contributed by PCRM nutrition director Amy Lanou, Ph.D.

Winter Vegetable Chowder

Serves 6

1 tsp canola oil
1/2 cup onion, chopped
1/2 cup celery, chopped
1 medium carrot, chopped
1 sweet potato, peeled and chopped
1 cup peeled, chopped butternut squash

(continued on next page)

(Winter Vegetable Chowder continued)

1/2 cup red bell pepper, chopped
1 tsp minced garlic
3 cups vegetable stock or water
1/2 tsp minced fresh thyme, or 1/4 tsp dried thyme leaves
2 cups kale, finely chopped
1 cup unsweetened soymilk
Salt and pepper to taste

Heat the oil in a large saucepan over medium heat and cook onions, celery and carrot for 5 minutes.

Add sweet potato, butternut squash, red bell pepper, garlic, stock or water, and thyme. Reduce heat and simmer for 20 minutes or until vegetables are tender.

Boil kale in lightly salted water for 5 minutes. Drain and set aside.

Purée soup in a blender until smooth. Return to saucepan. Stir in the soymilk, cooked kale and salt and pepper to taste. Slowly heat the soup, being very careful not to boil.

Recipe from 366 Simply Delicious Dairy Free Recipes *by Robin Robertson*

Salads

Asian Fusion Salad
Serves 8

A meal in itself!

1 head red leaf lettuce
1 heaping cup snow peas
1 large cucumber
1 sweet red pepper
1 1/2 cup bean sprouts
2 carrots
8 ounces flavored baked tofu (possible flavors: teriyaki, sesame, ginger, peanut, spicy Thai) or 1 15-ounce can white beans
1 tablespoon balsamic vinegar
1 teaspoon soy sauce
1 teaspoon sesame oil
1/4 teaspoon Thai chili paste or other chili sauce
low-fat salad dressing of your choice (possible flavors: sesame shiitake, tahini lemon, cilantro lime, etc.)

Wash and tear lettuce into bite-size pieces. Drain thoroughly and place in a large salad bowl. Trim tips from snow peas and cut on a diagonal into 1-inch slices. Peel cucumber, if desired, and julienne (cut into thin, narrow slices, 1 or 2 inches long). Cut red pepper in half and remove seeds and pith. Then, cut pepper into thin slices and cut slices diagonally into thirds. Rinse and drain bean sprouts. Julienne carrots and blanch them, if desired, by submerging them in boiling water for 3–4 minutes. Rinse with cold water and drain. Add snow peas, cucumber, red pepper, bean sprouts, and carrots to the salad, toss, and make an indentation in the center of the salad.

If using tofu, cut it into bite-sized pieces. If using beans, drain and rinse them. In a separate bowl, stir together vinegar, soy sauce, sesame oil, and chili paste. Pour over tofu or beans and toss. Add tofu or bean mixture to the center of the salad just before serving.

Serve with the salad dressing of your choice tossed in or on the side.

Recipe from PCRM Nutrition and Cooking Classes for Cancer Survivors;
contributed by PCRM nutrition director Amy Lanou, Ph.D.

Aztec Salad

Makes about 8 cups

This delicious salad is also a visual feast. It may be made in advance and keeps well for several days. The cilantro may be omitted if you prefer.

2 15-ounce cans black beans, drained and rinsed
1/2 cup finely chopped red onion
1 green bell pepper, seeded and diced
1 red or yellow bell pepper, seeded and diced
1 15-ounce can corn kernels, drained, or 1 10-ounce bag frozen corn, thawed, or 2 cups fresh corn
2 tomatoes, diced
3/4 cup chopped fresh cilantro *(optional)*
2 tablespoons seasoned rice vinegar
2 tablespoons apple cider or distilled vinegar
juice of 1 lemon or lime
2 garlic cloves, pressed or finely minced
2 teaspoons ground cumin
1 teaspoon coriander
1/2 teaspoon red pepper flakes or a pinch of cayenne

In a large bowl, combine beans, onion, bell peppers, corn, tomatoes, and cilantro (if using).

In a small bowl, whisk together vinegars, lemon or lime juice, garlic, cumin, coriander, and red pepper flakes. Pour over salad and toss gently to mix.

Recipe from Healthy Eating for Life to Prevent and Treat Diabetes *by Patricia Bertron, R.D.*

California Waldorf Salad

Makes about 6 cups

2 crisp, tangy apples (Fuji, winesap, Granny Smith, or similar)
1 large carrot, julienned or grated
1/2 cup raisins
1/4 cup chopped walnuts
1/3 cup vegan mayonnaise
3 tablespoons seasoned rice vinegar

Scrub and dice the apples, then place into a salad bowl. Add the carrots, raisins, walnuts, vegan mayonnaise, and vinegar. Stir to mix. Chill before serving, if possible.

Recipe from Healthy Eating for Life for Children *by Amy Lanou, Ph.D.*

Cucumber, Mango, and Spinach Salad

Serves 10 to 12

1 bag or bunch of spinach
1 mango, peeled and cut into bite size pieces
1 large English cucumber, peeled and sliced
6 scallions, thinly sliced
1/2 cup chopped fresh basil leaves
juice of 1 lime
1/2 cup seasoned rice vinegar
fresh cracked black pepper to taste

Wash and drain spinach, tear into bite-sized pieces if necessary, and put into a large serving bowl. Toss mango, cucumber, scallions, and basil in a medium bowl. Dress with lime juice and vinegar. Arrange mango mixture on spinach and sprinkle with fresh cracked black pepper.

Recipe from a PCRM Nutrition and Cooking Classes
for Cancer Survivors cooking demonstration

Easy Bean Salad

Serves 10

1/2 cup low-fat Italian salad dressing
1 15-ounce can kidney beans, drained and rinsed
1 15-ounce can pinto beans, drained and rinsed
1 15-ounce can black-eyed peas, drained and rinsed
1 10-ounce frozen package fordhook lima beans, thawed completely
1 cup frozen corn, thawed completely
1 large red bell pepper, diced
1/2 medium onion, diced
1 teaspoon salt
1 teaspoon pepper

Toss all ingredients together. Serve cold or at room temperature. May be covered and stored in the refrigerator for several days.

Recipe by PCRM dietitian Jennifer K. Reilly, R.D.

Fiesta Salad

Serves 10

This salad is a celebration of color and taste. It may be made in advance and keeps well for several days. If you are a cilantro lover, you may want to double the amount.

1 1/2 cups dry black beans, or 3 15-ounce cans black beans
3 1/2 cups water
(continued on next page)

2 cups frozen corn, thawed
2 large tomatoes, diced
1 large green bell pepper, diced
1 large red or yellow bell pepper, diced
1/2 cup chopped red onion
3/4 cup chopped cilantro *(optional)*
2 tablespoons seasoned rice vinegar
2 tablespoons apple cider or distilled vinegar
1 lime or lemon, juiced
2 garlic cloves, mined
2 teaspoons ground cumin
1 teaspoon ground coriander
1/2 teaspoon crushed red pepper, or a pinch of cayenne
1/2–1 teaspoon salt

If using dried beans, sort through beans to remove any debris, then wash them and place them in a large pan or bowl with about 6 cups water. Soak overnight. Pour off soaking water and place in a kettle with the 3 1/2 cups of fresh water. Bring to a simmer, and cook until the beans are just tender, about 45 minutes to 1 hour. (Although the beans should be thoroughly cooked, in this case they should not be overcooked.) Drain and cool the cooked beans. If using canned black beans, simply drain them and proceed.

When the beans are cool, combine them with the corn, tomatoes, bell peppers, red onion, and cilantro, if using. In a separate bowl, whisk together remaining ingredients and pour over the salad. Toss gently to mix.

Recipe from Food for Life *by Neal D. Barnard, M.D.;*
recipe by Jennifer Raymond

Fresh Spinach Salad

Serves 2

2 cups spinach
1/2 cup sliced mushrooms
1/4 cup chopped green onions
sea salt, to taste (optional)
tamari (optional)
sesame seeds for garnish

Thoroughly wash the spinach, tearing the larger leaves. Drain well. Add the mushrooms and green onions, and toss well. Sprinkle with tamari, if desired, then sprinkle each serving with sesame seeds.

Recipe from Vegetarian Cooking for People with Allergies
by Raphael Rettner, D.C.

Hoppin' John Salad

Makes about 5 cups

For the salad:
2 cups cooked black-eyed peas (1 cup dry) or 1 15-ounce can, drained
1 1/2 cups cooked brown rice (1/2 cup uncooked)
1/2 cup finely sliced green onions
1 celery stalk, thinly sliced (about 1/2 cup)
1 tomato, diced
2 tablespoon finely chopped parsley

For the vinaigrette:
1/4 cup lemon juice
1 tablespoon olive oil
1/4 teaspoon salt
1–2 garlic cloves, crushed

Combine the salad ingredients in a mixing bowl.

Mix together the vinaigrette ingredients and pour over salad. Toss gently. Chill 1 to 2 hours before serving if time permits.

Recipe from Turn Off the Fat Genes *by Neal D. Barnard, M.D.;*
recipe by Jennifer Raymond

Rootin' Tootin' Salad

Serves 6

Three root vegetables—beets, jicama, and carrots—combine to make this crunchy, nutritious salad.

1 15-ounce can diced beets, drained
1 small jicama, peeled and cut into thin strips or diced
2 medium carrots, peeled and cut into thin strips or diced
3 tablespoons of lemon juice
2 tablespoons seasoned rice vinegar
2 teaspoons stoneground mustard
1/2 teaspoon dried dill weed

Place beet cubes into a large salad bowl, along with jicama and carrot pieces. In a small bowl, mix lemon juice, vinegar, mustard, and dill; pour over the salad. Toss to mix. Serve warm or chilled.

Recipe from Foods That Fight Pain *by Neal Barnard, M.D.;*
recipe by Jennifer Raymond

Salad of Color

Serves 4

1 orange
1 sweet red pepper, cut into chunks
1 cup sugar snap peas, cut in half
1 cucumber, peeled and cut into chunks
8 fresh basil leaves, sliced
1 tablespoon seasoned rice vinegar
cracked black pepper, to taste

Peel the orange and cut the peeled fruit into bite-sized chunks. In a medium bowl, mix together the orange, red pepper, sugar snap peas, cucumber, and basil. Sprinkle with rice vinegar and season with pepper. Toss and serve.

Recipe from PCRM Weight Loss Study Cooking Demonstration;
contributed by PCRM nutrition director Amy Lanou, Ph.D.

Spinach Salad with Fruit Flavors

Serves 6

10 ounces chopped spinach, washed
1 cup berries or grapes or 10 strawberries, chopped
1 10-ounce can mandarin or clementine oranges, or grapefruit sections,
   drained & rinsed
1/4 cup sunflower seeds
1/4 cup chopped Brazil nuts
1/4 cup fat-free raspberry vinaigrette

Toss ingredients together and serve.

Stuffed Tomato Salad

Serves 5

5 large ripe tomatoes
1 can garbanzo beans (or 1 cup precooked chickpeas or garbanzo beans)
1 stalk celery, chopped *(optional)*
salt and pepper to taste

Scoop out tomatoes, saving pulp for a sauce. Fill tomatoes with beans and celery. Season with salt and pepper. Garnish with sauce and lettuce or sprouts.

Recipe from Meatless Meals for Working People
by Debra Wasserman and Charles Stahler

Tomato, Cucumber, and Basil Salad

Serves 6

4 fresh tomatoes, quartered and sliced
1/2 large English cucumber, peeled, quartered and sliced
1/2 cup fresh basil leaves,
3–4 tablespoons balsamic vinegar
fresh cracked black pepper, to taste

Arrange cucumber and tomato in a flat bowl. Add basil leaves, dress with balsamic vinegar, and sprinkle with fresh cracked black pepper.

Recipe by PCRM nutrition director Amy Lanou, Ph.D.

Side Dishes

Basic Brown Rice

Makes 3 cups

The addition of sea vegetables gives this brown rice an Asian flair. For plain brown rice, omit the sea salt and sea vegetables.

2 cups water
1 cup brown rice
1 teaspoon sea salt
1 strand kombu or several strands wakame

Bring the water to boil, and add the brown rice, sea salt, and sea vegetable. Return to a boil, lower the heat to a gentle simmer, cover, and cook 45 minutes.

Recipe from Vegetarian Cooking for People with Allergies
by Raphael Rettner, D.C.

Beets with Dill Sauce

Makes about 4 cups

4 medium beets
2 tablespoons lemon juice
1 tablespoon stone-ground mustard
1 tablespoon cider vinegar
1 tablespoon apple juice concentrate
1 teaspoon dried dill weed, or 1 tablespoon fresh dill, chopped

Wash and peel the beets, then slice them into 1/4-inch thick rounds. Steam over boiling water until tender when pierced with a fork, about 20 minutes. Mix the remaining ingredients in a serving bowl. Add the beets and toss to mix. Serve immediately, or chill before serving.

Recipe from Foods That Fight Pain *by Neal D. Barnard, M.D.;*
recipe by Jennifer Raymond

Braised Cabbage

Serves 2 to 3

1/2 cup water
2 cups coarsely chopped cabbage
salt
freshly ground black pepper
(continued on next page)

(Braised Cabbage continued)

Bring the water to a boil in a skillet or saucepan. Stir in the cabbage, cover, and cook until it is just tender, about 5 minutes. Sprinkle with salt and pepper to taste.

From Eat Right, Live Longer *by Neal D. Barnard, M.D.;*
recipe by Jennifer Raymond

Braised Collards or Kale

Makes 3 cups

Collard greens and kale are rich sources of calcium and beta-carotene, as well as other minerals and vitamins. One of the tastiest (and easiest) ways to prepare them is with a bit of soy sauce and plenty of garlic. Try to purchase young tender greens as these have the best flavor and texture.

1 bunch collard greens or kale (6–8 cups chopped)
1 teaspoon olive oil
2 teaspoons reduced-sodium soy sauce
1 teaspoon balsamic vinegar
2–3 garlic cloves, minced, or 2–3 teaspoons chopped
1/4 cup water

Wash greens, remove stems, then chop leaves into 1/2-inch wide strips. Combine olive oil, soy sauce, vinegar, garlic, and water in a large pot or skillet. Cook over high heat about 30 seconds. Reduce heat to medium-high, add chopped greens, and toss to mix. Cover and cook, stirring often, until greens are tender, about 5 minutes.

Recipe from Healthy Eating for Life for Children
by PCRM nutrition director Amy Lanou, Ph.D.

Broccoli with Sundried Tomatoes

Makes about 4 cups

The tangy flavor of sundried tomatoes is a perfect addition to steamed broccoli. Look for sundried tomatoes near the pickles and olives.

1 bunch broccoli
6 sundried tomatoes in olive oil, drained

Rinse broccoli and cut into florets. Peel and slice stems into rounds. Steam over boiling water until just tender, 3 to 5 minutes.

While broccoli is cooking, cut tomatoes into small pieces and place in a serving dish. When cooked, add broccoli to tomatoes, toss and serve.

Recipe from Healthy Eating for Life for Women *by Kristine Kieswer*

Calabacitas ("Little Squash")

Serves 4

This recipe came from a burrito shop in Ithaca, New York. It can be made with lima beans as well. It's a perfect vegetable combination for tostadas, tacos, or burritos, or it can be used as a side dish or as a baked potato topping. Since this recipe does not include any added sodium, add salt to tast if serving as a stand-alone side dish or potato topping.

1 small yellow onion, finely chopped
2 tablespoons water, divided
2 small zucchini, quartered lengthwise and sliced
8 ounces button mushrooms, sliced
1 1/2 cups frozen corn
1/2 teaspoon cumin
1/2 teaspoon chili powder

Braise onion in 1 tablespoon of the water, stirring until liquid has evaporated. Add sliced zucchini, mushrooms, and the remaining water. Stir in spices and simmer for 5 minutes, covered, until mushrooms are soft. Stir in corn and cook for 2 more minutes to heat through. Add black pepper to taste.

Recipe from PCRM Weight Loss Study Cooking Demonstration;
contributed by PCRM nutrition director Amy Lanou, Ph.D.

Collard Greens with Almonds

Serves 6

1/4 cup slivered almonds
1 pound collard greens, rinsed, thick stems removed
2 tablespoons toasted sesame oil
1 tablespoon rice vinegar
1 small garlic clove, minced

In a small skillet, toast almonds over medium heat until golden in color, 1 to 2 minutes; set aside.

Layer three collard leaves. Roll into cylinder and slice crosswise into thin strips. Repeat until all leaves are sliced. In large saucepan, bring 2 inches water to a boil over high heat. Add greens, cover, and steam 4 minutes.

In small bowl, whisk sesame oil, vinegar, and garlic until blended. Toss greens with dressing and garnish with toasted almonds. Serve hot.

Garlic Spinach

Serves 4

1 large bunch of fresh spinach
3 cloves of garlic
1 teaspoon vegetarian Worcestershire sauce
(continued on next page)

(Garlic Spinach continued)

Wash and de-stem spinach. Peel and mince garlic. Braise garlic in Worcestershire sauce over medium heat, stirring, until lightly browned. Add spinach to hot skillet. Use tongs to turn spinach until it is just wilted. Serve hot or at room temperature.

Recipe from PCRM Weight Loss Study Cooking Demonstration;
contributed by PCRM nutrition director Amy Lanou, Ph.D.

Hearty Barbecued Beans

Makes 6 cups

1 16-ounce can vegetarian baked beans
1 15-ounce can kidney beans
1 10-ounce package frozen baby lima beans
1 6-ounce can crushed tomatoes
1 cup finely chopped onion
1 tablespoon cider vinegar
1 tablespoon molasses
2 teaspoons stone-ground mustard
1 teaspoon chili powder

Combine all ingredients in a saucepan and cook at a slow simmer for 25 to 30 minutes.

Recipe from Turn Off the Fat Genes *by Neal D. Barnard, M.D.;*
recipe by Jennifer Raymond

Mashed Grains and Cauliflower

Serves 8

1 cup minced onion
1 teaspoon olive oil
2 cups millet, quinoa, couscous, or other grain of your choice
water for cooking 2 cups of selected grain according to package directions
4 cups cauliflower, cut into medium size pieces
1/2 teaspoon sea salt

Brush pot with oil and then add onion. Sauté for 3 minutes. Add grain and roast for 5 minutes. Add cauliflower, salt, and water. Cover pot and cook until grain has absorbed all the water. When the grains are done, mash the mixture together with a potato masher. Add a little water if necessary in order to get a smooth consistency. Serve topped with Mushroom Gravy (recipe on page 143).

Moroccan Carrots and Parsnips

Serves 6

1 teaspoon canola oil
3 tablespoons sweetener
1 1/2 teaspoons cinnamon
1/8 tsp cumin
1 3/4 cups orange juice
6 carrots, peeled and sliced
8 parsnips, peeled and sliced
1/2 cup chopped dried figs
1/4 cup raisins

In a large saucepan, heat oil over medium heat. Add sweetener, cinnamon, and cumin; cook, stirring for 1 minute. Add remaining ingredients and simmer, covered, for 25 minutes.

Adapted from Calci-Yum! *by David and Rachelle Bronfman*

Pan-Grilled Portabello Mushrooms

Serves 4

Serve with your favorite type of rice and a big pile of steamed spinach, chard, or collard greens. These mushrooms also work well as burgers in whole-grain buns with the desired condiments.

4 large portabello mushrooms
2 teaspoons olive oil
2 tablespoons red wine *(optional)*
2 tablespoons soy sauce
1 tablespoon balsamic vinegar
2 medium cloves garlic, minced, or 2 teaspoons chopped garlic

Clean mushrooms and trim stems flush with the bottom of the caps. In a large skillet, mix the remaining ingredients. Heat until the mixture begins to bubble; add mushrooms, tops down. Reduce to medium heat. Cover and cook for about 3 minutes, or until tops are browned. (If the pan becomes dry, add 2 to 3 tablespoons of water.) Turn the mushrooms and cook for about 5 minutes more, or until tender when pierced with a sharp knife. Serve hot.

Recipe from Foods That Fight Pain *by Neal Barnard, M.D.;
recipe by Jennifer Raymond*

Sautéed Broccoli with Ginger

Serves 4

1 clove garlic, minced
1/2-inch piece fresh ginger root, peeled and grated

(continued on next page)

(Sautéed Broccoli with Ginger continued)

2 teaspoons vegetable oil
1 pound broccoli, cut in florets
1 medium leek, sliced thin (white part only)
2 tablespoons vegetable stock
1 teaspoon tamari

Sauté the garlic and ginger in the oil in a large skillet for 1 minute. Add the broccoli, leek, and stock. Toss together all the ingredients to mix well. Cover the pan and cook for 3 minutes. Remove the cover and continue to sauté, stirring frequently, until the vegetables are just tender, about 10 minutes. Mix in the tamari and serve immediately.

Recipe from The Vegetarian Way, *by Virginia Messina, M.P.H., R.D., and Mark Messina, Ph.D.*

Spicy Black Beans and Tomatoes

Serves 4

1/4 cup vegetable broth
1/2 cup chopped onion
2 garlic cloves, minced
2 14.5-ounce cans diced tomatoes, drained
2 tablespoons canned chopped green chilies
2 15-ounce cans black beans, rinsed and drained
1 tablespoon chopped cilantro or parsley
1/2 teaspoon cumin
1/2 teaspoon ground red pepper
1/4 teaspoon chili powder

Heat vegetable broth in non-stick cooking skillet over medium-high heat. Add chopped onion and garlic; sauté in broth until tender. Add tomatoes and chilies. Reduce heat and cook, uncovered, 6 to 8 minutes or until mixture is slightly thickened, stirring occasionally. Stir in beans and remaining ingredients.

Cover and cook 5 minutes or until thoroughly heated. Serve over brown rice or cooked couscous, scoop up with baked tortilla chips, or wrap up in a tortilla to make a black bean burrito.

Recipe from PCRM Weight Loss Study Cooking Demonstration; contributed by PCRM dietitian Brie Turner-McGrievy, M.S., R.D.

Sure-Fire Roasted Vegetables

Vegetable Options
4 to 5 cups of "soft" veggies
- Chopped broccoli
- Chopped bell peppers
- Chopped zucchini or yellow summer squash
- Chopped eggplant

(continued on next page)

(Sure-Fire Roasted Vegetables continued)

OR

4 to 5 cups of "hard" veggies
   • Chopped carrots
   • Chopped sweet potatoes or new potatoes
   • Cubed butternut squash (or other squash)
   • Chopped parsnips or rutabaga
Onions and/or chopped garlic can be used with either soft or hard veggies.

Seasoning Mix Options
Italian:
   • 2 teaspoons dried basil
   • 1 teaspoon dried oregano
   • 2 teaspoons dried rosemary
   • 1/4 teaspoon salt
   • 1/4 teaspoon pepper
   • 1/4 cup chopped fresh parsley
Mexican:
   • 2 teaspoons cumin
   • 1 teaspoon basil
   • 1 teaspoon rosemary
   • 1/4 teaspoon salt
   • 1/4 teaspoon pepper
   • 1/4 cup chopped cilantro
Indian:
   • 1 teaspoon curry powder
   • 1 teaspoon garam masala
   • 1/4 teaspoon salt
   • 1/4 teaspoon pepper
   • 1/4 cup chopped cilantro

Preheat oven to 400°F. Spray jelly roll pan with cooking spray.

Combine vegetable mixture (either hard or soft vegetables) in bowl. Add your choice of seasoning mix. Toss vegetables to coat with seasoning. Place vegetables in pan in a single layer.

For *soft* vegetables: Roast 10 minutes. Take pan out of oven and spray the tops of the vegetables with cooking spray. Turn veggies and cook for another 5 to 10 minutes or until vegetables are tender.

For *hard* vegetables: Roast 15 minutes. Take pan out of oven and spray the tops of the vegetables with cooking spray. Turn veggies and cook for another 15 minutes or until vegetables are tender.

Make it a meal by adding a can of drained and rinsed beans (such as garbanzo or black beans). Serve vegetables as a side dish, over couscous or brown rice, or wrapped up in a burrito with salsa.

Recipe from PCRM Weight Loss Study Cooking Demonstration;
contributed by PCRM dietitian Brie Turner-McGrievy, R.D.

Three Bean Delight

Serves 4

1 cup cooked kidney beans
1 cup cooked garbanzo beans
1 cup cooked lima beans
1 cup onion, chopped
1/2 cup green pepper, chopped
4 teaspoons olive oil

Toss all ingredients together. Serve hot or cold with a grain or bread. To serve cold for a salad, add a few drops of lemon juice or vinegar.

Recipe from Vegetarian Cooking for People with Diabetes
by Patricia Le Shane

Wonderful Winter Squash

Makes 4 cups

1 medium winter squash (butternut or kabocha, for example)
1/2 cup water
2 teaspoons soy sauce
2 tablespoons maple syrup

Slice the squash in half, then peel and remove the seeds. Cut the squash into 1-inch cubes (you should have about 4 cups).

Place the cubes in a large pot with the water. Add the soy sauce and syrup. Cover and simmer over medium heat for 15 to 20 minutes or until squash is tender when pierced with a fork.

Recipe from Foods That Fight Pain *by Neal Barnard, M.D.;*
recipe by Jennifer Raymond

Zippy Yams and Collards

Serves 4

1 bunch collards, finely sliced
2 small yams, cut into bite-sized chunks
1 onion, sliced
2 large cloves of garlic, minced
1 tablespoon vegetarian Worcestershire sauce
1/2 teaspoon Thai chili paste
1/2 lemon

Put yams in a deep skillet and just cover them with water. Cover skillet and boil yams for 5 to 10 minutes until soft when pierced with a fork. Add onions and garlic and continue to simmer until about half of the water has boiled away. Add vegetarian Worcestershire sauce, chili paste, and collards. Simmer until the collards are soft. Squeeze lemon over the mixture and serve.

Zucchini Skillet Hash

Serves 8

8 ounces gluten-free pasta (quinoa, rice, etc.)
1/2 cup water
1 medium onion, chopped
2 medium stalks celery, sliced thin
2 medium zucchinis, diced
3 vegan burger patties, chopped
1 15-ounce can garbanzo beans, including liquid
1/2 teaspoon salt

Cook pasta according to package directions. Drain and rinse, then set aside. In a large skillet, heat the water; add onion and garlic. Cook over high heat for about 3 minutes or until onion is soft. Add mushrooms and celery and continue cooking, stirring frequently, for about 5 minutes or until the mushrooms begin to brown. Add burger patties and cook, stirring often, for about 3 minutes, or until zucchini is just tender when pierced with a fork.

Purée beans, with their liquid, in a blender or food processor. Add to the vegetable mixture, along with pasta and salt. Heat gently, stirring frequently, until hot and steamy.

Recipe from Foods That Fight Pain *by Neal D. Barnard, M.D.;*
recipe by Jennifer Raymond

Sandwiches and Wraps

Missing Egg Sandwich

Serves 6

These sandwiches have the flavor and appearance of egg salad without the saturated fat and cholesterol.

1/2 pound firm reduced-fat tofu (1 cup)
1 green onion, finely chopped, including green top
2 tablespoons pickle relish
2 tablespoons vegan mayonnaise
2 teaspoons stone-ground mustard
2 teaspoons reduced-sodium soy sauce
1/4 teaspoon cumin
1/4 teaspoon turmeric
1/4 teaspoon garlic powder
12 slices whole-grain bread
6 lettuce leaves
6 tomato slices

Mash tofu, leaving some chunks. Add green onion, pickle relish, vegan mayonnaise, mustard, soy sauce, cumin, turmeric, and garlic powder. Mix well. Spread on whole-grain bread and garnish with lettuce and tomato slices.

Recipe from Healthy Eating for Life for Children *by Amy Lanou, Ph.D.*

Submarine Sandwiches

Serves 4

1 pound baked tofu
4 submarine sandwich rolls
sliced onion
sliced green pepper
sliced tomato
lettuce leaves
pickles
1 tablespoon herb-flavored vinegar
2 tablespoons olive oil

(continued on next page)

(Submarine Sandwiches continued)

Slice the baked tofu and spread slices in each of the rolls. Top with slices of vegetables. Whisk together the vinegar and oil and drizzle just a small amount into each sandwich.

Recipe from The Vegetarian No-Cholesterol Family-Style Cookbook
by Kate Schumann and Virginia Messina, M.P.H., R.D.

Thai Wraps

Serves 6

1 tablespoon peanut butter
3 tablespoons water
2 tablespoons soy sauce
1 small onion, chopped
1 carrot, thinly sliced
1 celery stalk, thinly sliced
2 cups sliced mushrooms
1/2 pound firm tofu, cut into 1/2-inch cubes
1 1/2 teaspoons curry powder
1/2 red bell pepper, diced
1/2 cup chopped cilantro *(optional)*
2 cups finely chopped kale
6 large flour tortillas
2 cups cooked brown rice
6 tablespoons Plum Sauce (recipe follows)

Mix the peanut butter with 3 tablespoons of water. Set aside.

Heat 1/2 cup of water and the soy sauce in a large, nonstick skillet. Add the onion, carrot, celery, and mushrooms, and cook 5 minutes, stirring occasionally. Stir in the tofu and cook over medium-high heat, stirring often, until the vegetables are tender, about 5 minutes. Stir in the curry powder, red bell pepper, cilantro (if using), kale, and peanut butter mixture. Cover and cook until the kale is tender, about 5 minutes.

Heat the tortillas in a dry skillet until soft. Place about 1/2 cup of the vegetable mixture along the center of the tortilla. Top with 1/3 cup of brown rice and 2 teaspoons of Plum Sauce. Roll the tortilla around the filling.

Plum Sauce:
1 17-ounce can purple plums in heavy syrup
2 garlic cloves
1 tablespoon cornstarch
2 tablespoons seasoned rice vinegar
1 tablespoon soy sauce
1/8 teaspoon cayenne (more or less to taste)

(continued on next page)

(Thai Wraps continued)

Remove pits from the plums, then purée plums in a blender or food processor along with their liquid and the remaining ingredients. Heat in a saucepan, stirring constantly, until thickened.

Recipe from Turn Off the Fat Genes *by Neal Barnard, M.D.;*
recipe by Jennifer Raymond

Veggie Wraps

Makes 4 wraps

Veggie Wraps make a perfectly delicious, vegetable-rich meal.

1/4 cup sunflower seeds
4 whole wheat tortillas
1–2 cups hummus
1–2 cups mixed salad greens or torn leaf lettuce
1 carrot, shredded
1 cup bean sprouts

Preheat oven or toaster oven to 375°F.

Place sunflower seeds in a small ovenproof dish and oven-roast until lightly browned and fragrant, about 10 minutes. Set aside.

Warm tortillas, one at a time, in a large, dry skillet, flipping to warm both sides until soft and pliable.

Spread each tortilla evenly with about 1/2 cup of hummus, leaving edges uncovered.

Divide remaining ingredients evenly among tortillas.

Wrap tortillas around filling.

Recipe from Healthy Eating for Life for Women *by Kristine Kieswer*

Main Dishes

Beet This Burger

Serves 6

This burger comes from Olinda Cho-Forsythe, a native of Guatemala and a full-blooded Mayan. She developed her burger recipe in the kitchens of the Gran Fraternidad Universal, an organization dedicated to world peace and to promoting a vegetarian diet through its centers and restaurants throughout Latin America. The unusual addition of 1 tablespoon of grated beets is just enough to give this burger a pleasant color.

1 tablespoon finely grated raw beet
1/2 cup cooked oats
1 cup uncooked oats
1/2 cup coarsely ground walnuts
1/4 cup coarsely ground almonds
2 tablespoons sesame seeds
1 tablespoon nutritional yeast flakes *(optional)*
1/4 cup minced green pepper
1/4 cup minced onion
1 teaspoon dried basil
1/4 teaspoon dried thyme
1/4 teaspoon ground sage
1/4 teaspoon mustard powder
2 tablespoons soy sauce
1 tablespoon instant dry vegetable broth
tomato slices for garnish

Mix all ingredients (except tomato slices) together well. Form into 6 patties and grill until cooked through. Serve on whole-wheat rolls with tomato slices and your favorite condiments.

Recipe from The Vegetarian No-Cholesterol Barbecue Cookbook
by Kate Schumann and Virginina Messina, M.P.H., R.D.

Black Bean Pueblo Pie

Makes a generous 9×13-inch casserole (12 servings)

This is like a lasagna with a Southwestern twist. It is layered with black bean chili, corn tortillas, spicy tomato sauce, and tangy garbanzo spread.

Beans:
4 cups cooked black beans (or 2 15-ounce cans)
1 15-ounce can crushed tomatoes
1/2 cup water
2 teaspoons paprika
2 teaspoons chili powder
2 teaspoons onion powder
1 teaspoon garlic powder

Tomato Sauce:
1 large onion, chopped
1 tablespoon minced garlic (about 4 large cloves)
1 28-ounce can crushed tomatoes
4 teaspoons chili powder
2 teaspoons cumin

Garbanzo spread:
1 15-ounce can garbanzo beans, drained
1/2 cup water-packed roasted red pepper (about 2 peppers)
2 garlic cloves, peeled
1 tablespoon tahini (sesame seed butter)
3 tablespoons lemon juice
1/2 teaspoon cumin

4–6 corn tortillas, torn in half
1 cup chopped green onions

Combine black beans, crushed tomatoes, water, paprika, chili powder, onion powder, and garlic powder in a pot. Bring to a simmer, then cover and cook, stirring frequently, for 25 minutes.

To make sauce, heat 1/2 cup of water in a large pot or skillet. Cook onion and garlic over high heat, stirring often, until soft, about 5 minutes. Add tomatoes, chili powder, and cumin. Cover and simmer over medium heat 5 minutes.

Combine garbanzo beans, roasted peppers, garlic, tahini, and lemon juice in a food processor or blender. Process until very smooth, about 2 minutes.

Preheat oven to 350°F.

Spread 1/2 to 1 cup of the tomato sauce in a 9×13-inch (or larger) baking dish. Cover with a layer of tortillas, then spread with half of the garbanzo spread, using your fingers to hold tortillas in place. Sprinkle with half of the black beans and green onions. Top with half of the tomato sauce.

Repeat layers, ending with tomato sauce. Bake in preheated oven for 25 minutes.

Recipe from Healthy Eating for Life to Prevent and Treat Cancer *by Vesanto Melina, M.S., R.D.*

Brussels Sprouts with Udon Noodles in a Miso Sauce

Serves 6

1 pound Brussels sprouts
1 teaspoon olive oil
1 tablespoon fresh ginger, minced
2 cloves garlic, minced
6 scallions, thinly sliced (keep white and green parts separate)
1 red pepper, finely diced
1 yellow or purple pepper, finely diced
1/4–1/2 teaspoon crushed red pepper flakes
3/4 cup water
8 ounces udon noodles, prepared according to package directions (al dente)
2 1/2 tablespoons dark miso, dissolved in 1/2 cup warm water (use
   noodle water)
1–2 tablespoons low-sodium tamari

Trim off root end of Brussels sprouts and discard any damaged outer leaves. Cut Brussels sprouts into 1/4-inch slices.

In a large skillet, heat the oil over medium heat. Add the ginger and garlic, and sauté for 20 seconds. Add the white part of the scallions, peppers, and red pepper flakes, and cook, stirring constantly, for one minute.

Turn off the heat. Add Brussels sprouts and water (be careful of splattering oil). Return to medium heat and cook until Brussels sprouts are tender-crisp, 4 to 5 minutes.

Add prepared udon noodles to skillet with Brussels sprouts. Stir in miso sauce, reserved scallions and tamari. Cook until well heated and serve immediately.

Recipe adapted from The New Vegan Cookbook *by Lorna Sass*

Buckwheat Pasta with Seitan

Serves 6

Seitan is a high-protein wheat product with a meaty taste and texture. In this recipe, it is served with soba, Japanese buckwheat pasta. Look for seitan in health food stores. Soba is available in the Asian food section of many supermarkets and health food stores, as well as in Asian markets.

1 medium onion, chopped
2 tablespoons oil
3 cups sliced fresh mushrooms
8 ounces seitan, sliced
2 tablespoons flour
1 1/2 cups cold water
2 teaspoons soy sauce
1/2 teaspoon garlic powder, or 1 teaspoon chopped garlic

(continued on next page)

(Buckwheat Pasta with Seitan continued)

1/4 teaspoon black pepper
12 ounces soba noodles
1 teaspoon salt

Sauté the onion in a large skillet with the oil until transparent, then add the mushrooms.

Cover and continue cooking until mushrooms are brown, then stir in the seitan.

Whisk flour and water together until smooth, then add to the skillet along with the soy sauce, garlic powder, and pepper. Cook, uncovered, over medium-low heat until thickened.

Meanwhile, bring water to boil in a separate pasta pot. Add the soba noodles and the salt and boil until al dente, about 8 minutes. Top with seitan mixture and serve.

Recipe from Food for Life *by Neal D. Barnard, M.D.;*
recipe by Jennifer Raymond

Creamy Veggie Curry

Makes 4 servings

Rich and full of flavor, this dish is best when served over brown rice.

1 large onion, sliced
4 cloves garlic, minced, or 4 teaspoons chopped
3 large carrots, diced
2 tablespoons canola oil
1 medium potato, cubed
1 1/2 cups cauliflower florets, chopped, or 1 bag frozen chopped cauliflower florets
1 cup broccoli florets, chopped, or 1 bag frozen chopped broccoli florets
8 mushrooms, sliced
1 can chickpeas, drained and rinsed
1 1/2 tablespoons curry powder
1 teaspoon cumin
1/2 teaspoon turmeric
pinch of cayenne pepper
1 cup reduced-fat coconut milk or soymilk
1 cup fresh or frozen peas
3 tablespoons lite soy sauce

In a large saucepan, sauté the onions, garlic, and carrots in oil on medium-high heat until the onions become translucent. Add the remaining vegetables, chickpeas, curry, cumin, turmeric, and cayenne, cooking for 2–4 minutes and stirring often so they don't stick to the pan. Add the coconut milk or soymilk, cover, and reduce the heat to medium-low. Simmer for
(continued on next page)

(Creamy Veggie Curry continued)

10–20 minutes, stirring occasionally, until potatoes can be pierced easily with a fork. Stir in the peas and soy sauce, and cook uncovered on medium-high heat, stirring constantly, until the liquid has thickened. Serve over rice or noodles.

Note: You can use whatever vegetables you have around (e.g., spinach, kale, green onions).

Recipe adapted from How It All Vegan!
by Tanya Barnard and Sarah Kramer

Easy Stir-Fry

Serves 4

1 bag "Create A Meal" frozen mixed vegetables or 1 bag frozen stir-fry
   vegetables plus 1/4 cup low-fat stir-fry sauce
1 package teriyaki-flavored faux chicken strips or 1 can of your favorite
   beans, drained and rinsed

Follow directions on package, substituting beans or meat alternative for the suggested beef, chicken, or fish. To reduce the sodium content, use only 1/2 of the sauce package.

Serve over couscous, brown rice, or your favorite whole grain.

Recipe from a PCRM Weight Loss Study Cooking Demonstration;
contributed by PCRM dietitian Brie Turner-McGrievy, M.S., R.D.

Greens and Grains Croquettes

Makes 15 to 18 patties

1 cup dry quinoa, cooked according to package directions with water or
vegetable stock
15-ounce block soft tofu, mashed
1 bunch collard greens, washed, finely chopped, and boiled for 3–5 minutes
1/2 onion, minced
1/2 cup ground almonds
2 teaspoons Italian seasoning
1 teaspoon salt
1 teaspoon pepper
flour for shaping and dredging
canola or olive oil for brushing

Preheat oven to 350°F.

Combine tofu with quinoa. Add collards, onions, almonds, Italian seasoning, and salt and pepper, mixing by hand. Form into 15–18 patties; chill well.

Dredge patties in flour. Brush croquettes with olive oil and place on a light-
(continued on next page)

ly oiled baking tray. Bake for 15 minutes, turn the croquettes over, brush with oil, and bake for another 10–12 minutes. Or, pan-fry on each side in a little bit of oil until crispy.

Homestyle Squash and Pinto Beans

Serves 4

Veggies, rice, and beans make this all-American dish a welcome guest after a hard day. Serve with a salad and fruit wedges.

1/4 cup vegetable broth (or more as needed for sauté)
1/2 cup chopped onion
2 teaspoons seeded, minced jalapeño pepper
2 garlic cloves, minced
1 cup (1/2-inch-thick) sliced yellow squash
1 cup (1/2-inch-thick) sliced zucchini
1/2 cup fresh corn kernels
1 16-ounce can pinto beans, drained
1 14.5-ounce can diced tomatoes, undrained
3 thyme sprigs
2 cups hot cooked brown rice

Heat broth in a large skillet over medium-high heat. Add the onion, jalapeno, and garlic, and sauté 2 minutes. Stir in squash and zucchini, and sauté 2 minutes. Add corn, beans, tomatoes, and thyme; cover, reduce heat, and simmer 10 minutes. Discard thyme sprigs.

Serve over rice.

Indian Split Pea Dahl

Serves 6

1 1/2 cups yellow split peas
3 cups water
1 large onion, chopped
1 small green pepper, chopped
1 teaspoon turmeric
1/2 teaspoon curry powder
1 1/2 teaspoon black mustard seeds
1/2 cup water
juice of 1 lemon
salt to taste

Simmer split peas in 3 cups water for 30 minutes or until tender. Add more water, if needed.

(continued on next page)

(Indian Split Pea Dahl continued)

In another saucepan, simmer chopped onions, green peppers, turmeric, curry powder, mustard seeds, and water for 15 minutes or until onions and peppers are tender. Mix with peas and add lemon juice and salt.

Serve over a generous portion of brown rice. Chutney is a nice accompaniment.

Recipe from The Power of Your Plate *by Neal Barnard, M.D.*

Neat Loaf

Makes one loaf (about 12 slices)

1 cup cooked brown rice
2 cups bread crumbs
1 cup finely chopped walnuts
1 small onion, finely chopped
2 celery stalks, finely chopped
1 carrot, finely chopped
1 pound firm tofu
1/4 cup barbecue sauce
3 tablespoons reduced-sodium soy sauce
2 teaspoons stone-ground or Dijon mustard
1/4 teaspoon black pepper
barbecue sauce or ketchup for topping

Preheat oven to 350°F.

In a large bowl, combine the brown rice, bread crumbs, walnuts, onion, celery, and carrot.

Purée the tofu in a food processor or mash by hand until very smooth. Add to the rice mixture along with the barbecue sauce, soy sauce, mustard, and black pepper.

Stir with a large spoon or knead mixture by hand until it is well mixed and holds together, about 1 minute.

Transfer to an oil-sprayed 5- x 9-inch loaf pan or other baking dish and distribute evenly using a spoon, spatula, or your hand.

Top with barbecue sauce or ketchup. Bake 60 minutes. Let stand 10 minutes before serving.

Recipe from Healthy Eating for Life for Children *by Amy Lanou, Ph.D.*

New Year's Day Hoppin' John

Serves 4

3 cups cooked long-grain rice
2 15-ounce cans black-eyed peas
1 cup chopped red onion
1 clove garlic, minced
1 cup chopped celery
2 tablespoons chopped fresh parsley
1 teaspoon salt
1/2 teaspoon black pepper
dash of hot sauce

Preheat oven to 350° F.

Combine all ingredients in a casserole dish coated with cooking spray.

Bake uncovered for 20 minutes or until thoroughly heated.

*Recipe from a PCRM Weight Loss Study Cooking Demonstration;
contributed by PCRM dietitian Brie Turner-McGrievy, M.S., R.D.*

Pasta con Asparagi

Serves 4

Maria D'Orazio brought her culinary genius and Italy's warmest smile to
Toronto. In this dish, she combines two favorites. We have lightened the
recipe by sautéing with water or vegetable stock instead of oil.

1 to 2 tablespoons water or vegetable stock
1 medium onion, chopped
1 28-ounce can tomatoes, chopped
2 pounds fresh asparagus
1 tablespoon chopped fresh basil
1/4 teaspoon ground sage
8 ounces spaghetti

Heat water or vegetable stock in a large nonstick pan. Add onion and
sauté over medium heat for 3 minutes, until translucent. Add tomatoes,
asparagus, basil, and sage. Bring to a boil, cover, and simmer for 7 minutes.
Remove from heat and keep warm.

Cook pasta according to package directions, omitting any fat or salt. Drain
pasta and place in a serving bowl. Add the asparagus mixture and toss.
Serve immediately.

Tip: Because asparagus tips cook faster than the thicker ends, you may
wish to thin the asparagus with a potato peeler or chop off the ends.

Recipe from Solo Maria, Toronto, Canada, printed in
The Best in the World *edited by Neal Barnard, M.D.*

Penne with Fresh Spinach, Tomatoes, and Olives

Serves 4

1 tablespoon olive oil
1 medium onion, chopped
2 14.5-ounce cans chopped tomatoes
1/2 cup kalamata olives, pitted and sliced
1 pound fresh spinach, coarsely chopped
1/2 cup chopped fresh parsley
8 ounces penne pasta
1/4 cup vegan parmesan cheese or nutritional yeast *(optional)*

Heat oil in a large, nonstick skillet. Add onion and sauté over medium heat for 3 minutes. Add chopped tomatoes. Bring to a boil and then reduce heat, cover, and simmer for 20 minutes. Add sliced olives, chopped spinach, and parsley. Cook an additional 5 minutes.

Meanwhile, cook pasta according to package directions, omitting any fat or salt. Drain and transfer to a serving bowl. Add spinach mixture and toss gently. Serve immediately. Sprinkle vegan parmesan or nutritional yeast over top, if desired.

Recipe from The Best in the World, *edited by Neal D. Barnard, M.D.*

Quick Bean Burritos

Serves 4

4 fat-free flour or corn tortillas
1 15-ounce can fat-free refried beans
1 cup shredded romaine lettuce
2 medium green onions, sliced
1/2 cup Tomato Corn Salsa (page 85) or other favorite salsa
1/2 cup Guacamole Plus (page 83) or Mockamole (page 84)

Heat beans in small saucepan or in microwave until warmed through. In a large skillet, heat a tortilla until it is warm and soft, or warm tortillas in the microwave if making more than 4 tortillas. Spread about 1/2 cup of the beans down the center, then top with lettuce, green onions, salsa, and, if using, the guacamole. Fold the bottom end toward the center, then roll the tortilla around the filling. Repeat with remaining tortillas or let those dining make their own.

Recipe adapted from Foods That Fight Pain *by Neal Barnard, M.D.;*
recipe by Jennifer Raymond

Quickie Quesadillas

Makes 8 quesadillas

These quesadillas are a truly happy marriage between cultures: Middle

(continued on next page)

(Quickie Quesadillas continued)
Eastern red pepper hummus warmed in corn tortillas and garnished with salsa makes an absolutely delicious meal or snack.

1 15-ounce can garbanzo beans
1/2 cup water-packed roasted red pepper
3 tablespoons lemon juice
1 tablespoon tahini (sesame seed butter)
1 garlic clove, peeled
1/4 teaspoon cumin
8 corn tortillas
1/2 cup chopped green onions
1/2–1 cup salsa

Drain garbanzo beans and place in a food processor or blender with roasted peppers, lemon juice, tahini, garlic, and cumin. Process until very smooth, 1–2 minutes.

Spread a tortilla with 2–3 tablespoons of garbanzo mixture and place in a large non-stick skillet over medium heat. Sprinkle with chopped green onions and salsa.

Top with a second tortilla and cook until the bottom tortilla is warm and soft, 2–3 minutes. Turn and cook the second side for another minute. Remove from pan and cut in half. Repeat with remaining tortillas.

Recipe from Healthy Eating for Life for Children *by Amy Lanou, Ph.D.*

Sesame Bok Choy and Carrot Stir-Fry

Serves 2

This recipe is delicious served over quinoa, brown rice, or other whole grain. But it can also be served alone as a vegetable side dish.

1 teaspoon dark sesame oil
4 cloves garlic, minced
3 carrots, cut diagonally into 1/4-inch slices
1/2 cup chopped green onions
5 cups bok choy, cut into 1/2-inch pieces
1/4 cup vegetable stock
2 teaspoons minced ginger root
1 teaspoon granulated sugar
2 tablespoons toasted sesame seeds
3 cups cooked quinoa or other whole grain

In a large nonstick skillet or wok, heat oil over medium heat. Add garlic, carrots and green onions; stir-fry for 3 minutes. Add bok choy and stir-fry another 2 minutes. Stir in vegetable stock, ginger, and sugar. Reduce heat and simmer 5 minutes.

Sprinkle sesame seeds over stir-fry. Spoon over quinoa or other whole grain.

Recipe from CalciYum! *by David and Rachelle Bronfman*

Spaghetti Balls

Makes 36 balls

Pour 1 3/4 cups boiling water over 2 cups dry textured vegetable protein and soak for 10 minutes.

Steam together for a few minutes:
1/2 cup water
1 small onion, diced

Mix onion with textured vegetable protein and stir in:
1/2 cup unbleached flour
1 teaspoon salt
1 tablespoon low-sodium soy sauce
1/2 teaspoon chili powder
1/2 teaspoon garlic powder
1/2 teaspoon oregano

Shape this mixture into balls one inch in diameter, pressing firmly. Spray vegetable oil into a non-stick pan and cook balls until browned. Or shape into patties, fry lightly until brown, and serve in buns.

Recipe from The Power of Your Plate *by Neal D. Barnard, M.D.*

Spicy Thai Peanut Satay

Serves 5 to 8

No, it's not from Thailand; it's from Wisconsin. The Ovens on Monroe Street is a bakery and restaurant featuring delightful dishes, this one in the Thai tradition.

4 cups vegetables, fruits, and nuts (use any combination of broccoli, carrots, cauliflower, red cabbage, green peppers, scallions, tomatoes, mushrooms, unsalted cashew halves, cilantro, raisins, and pineapple chunks totaling 4 cups)
1 tablespoon water
1 tablespoon minced garlic
1 tablespoon olive oil

Sauté the vegetable/fruit/nut mixture with the water, garlic, and olive oil. Serve over rice topped with Peanut Sauce (recipe follows).

Peanut Sauce:
Serves 5 to 8
1/4 cup soy sauce
1 cup peanut butter
2 tablespoons minced fresh garlic
1 tablespoon red curry paste
1/4 cup water
1/4 cup cooking sherry

(continued on next page)

(Spicy Thai Peanut Satay continued)

2 to 3 dashes of Tabasco
1 cup lemon or lime juice
1/2 teaspoon cayenne
1/2 tablespoon onion powder
1/2 tablespoon basil
1/4 teaspoon paprika
salt and pepper to taste

Mix all ingredients, using a whisk or blender, until creamy.

Recipe from The Ovens on Monroe Street, Madison, Wisconsin, printed in
The Best in the World, *edited by Neal Barnard, M.D.*

Tamale Pie

Serves 8

This simple, satisfying casserole has vegetarian chili on the bottom and cornbread on the top.

2 cups soymilk
2 tablespoons vinegar
6 cups vegetarian chili (canned or homemade)
2 cups cornmeal
2 teaspoons baking soda
1/2 teaspoon salt
2 tablespoons oil

Preheat oven to 400°F.

Combine the soymilk and vinegar and let stand 5 minutes or more.

Meanwhile, heat the chili until very hot, then pour into a 9×12-inch baking dish.

Mix the cornmeal, baking soda, and salt in a large bowl, then add the soymilk mixture and oil. Stir just to mix, then pour over the hot chili, and bake until the bread is set and golden brown, about 30 minutes.

Recipe from Food for Life *by Neal D. Barnard, M.D.;*
recipe by Jennifer Raymond

Taste of Morocco

Serves 4

Hearty enough to feed a tribe of hungry Bedouins—or teeny boppers. Using frozen peppers cuts the cooking time to about 20 minutes.

1 zucchini, cubed
1 sweet potato or small winter squash, cubed
(continued on next page)

(Taste of Morocco continued)
1 clove garlic, minced or pressed
1 tablespoon oil
1/4 cup water
1 15-ounce can chickpeas
1 teaspoon ground cumin
1/2 teaspoon allspice
1/2 teaspoon ground ginger
1/2 teaspoon turmeric
1/2 teaspoon paprika
1/4 teaspoon salt
1/4 teaspoon cayenne
1/4 teaspoon cinnamon
1 red bell pepper, diced
1 yellow bell pepper, diced
2 cups uncooked couscous
1/2 cup raisins

Sauté the zucchini, sweet potato or squash, and garlic in the oil until partially cooked, about 5 minutes. Use water as necessary to keep the vegetables from sticking. Drain and rinse the chickpeas. Add the seasonings, chickpeas, and peppers to the pan. Cover and cook for about 5 minutes.

Meanwhile, place the couscous and raisins in another saucepan. Add enough water so that the couscous is covered by about 1/2 inch. Bring the mixture to a boil, then cover tightly, remove from the heat, and let stand for at least 10 minutes. Remove the cover from the pepper/chickpea mixture, stir, and cook a few minutes longer to heat thoroughly and thicken. Serve the bean and pepper stew over the couscous.

Recipe from Cooking with PETA *by People for the Ethical Treatment of Animals*

Tempeh and Eggplant Pot Pies
Serves 2

Chunky, individual vegetable pies topped with a biscuit-style crust—honest food at its robust best.

Filling:
2 cups eggplant, diced (about 1 very small Western eggplant or 1 to 2 Asian eggplants)
1 8-ounce can tomato sauce (1 cup)
1/2 cup onion, chopped
1/2 cup celery, chopped
4 ounces (1/4 pound) tempeh, cut into 1/2-inch cubes
1 teaspoon olive oil (optional)
salt and pepper to taste
(continued on next page)

(Tempeh and Eggplant Pot Pies continued)
Biscuit Crust:
1/2 cup whole wheat pastry flour
1 teaspoon non-aluminum baking powder (such as Rumford)
1/4 cup water
2 teaspoons olive oil
pinch of salt

Preheat the oven to 350°F. Coat two 15-ounce or 16-ounce individual casserole dishes with nonstick cooking spray, and set them aside.

To make the filling, place all the filling ingredients except the salt and pepper in a 4 1/2-quart saucepan or Dutch oven. Place the saucepan over high heat, and bring the mixture to a boil. Reduce the heat to medium, cover the saucepan with a lid, and simmer the mixture, stirring once or twice, for 15 minutes.

Remove the saucepan from the heat and season the filling with salt and pepper to taste.

Divide the filling evenly between the prepared casserole dishes, and set aside.

To prepare the biscuit crust, place the flour, baking powder, and salt in a small mixing bowl, and stir them together. Pour the water and oil into the flour mixture at the same time, and mix just until the dry ingredients are evenly moistened. The dough will be stiff.

Drop the dough by 4 small spoonfuls on top of each casserole (2 per casserole). Then carefully spread the dough out with the back of the spoon so it evenly covers the top of the filling.

Bake the pot pies until the crust is golden, about 20 to 25 minutes. Serve hot.

Recipe from Table for Two: Meat- and Dairy-Free Recipes *by Joanne Stepaniak*

Tempeh Broccoli Sauté

Serves 4

1 10-ounce package tempeh, cubed
2 stalks broccoli, chopped, or 2 bags frozen broccoli florets
1 small onion, minced
1 red bell pepper, chopped
1 teaspoon powdered or fresh ginger
1 tablespoon chopped garlic
2 tablespoons oil
1 tablespoon tamari or soy sauce

Cube tempeh into ½-inch pieces and steam in water for 10 minutes. Discard cooking water. Sauté cubed tempeh, broccoli, onion, and red pepper with garlic and ginger in oil over medium-high heat until tempeh is lightly browned. Add soy sauce at last moment. Serve with brown rice.

Recipe adapted from Simply Vegan *by Debra Wasserman*

Tempeh with Apricot Marinade

Serves 8

1 pound tempeh
1 cup apricot preserves
1 clove garlic, peeled and minced
2 tablespoons oil
1/4 cup soy sauce
2 tablespoons cider vinegar

Cut the tempeh into 2-inch squares. Place in a vegetable steamer and steam for 20 minutes.

Combine the apricot preserves, garlic, oil, soy sauce, and vinegar and mix thoroughly. Place the steamed tempeh in a large bowl and pour the apricot marinade over it. Marinate in the refrigerator for an hour.

Grill, brushing frequently with the marinade and turning the tempeh pieces every few minutes, until tempeh is browned and completely heated through. Serve on rolls or over rice.

Recipe from The Vegetarian No-Cholesterol Barbecue Cookbook
by Kate Schumann and Virginia Messina, M.P.H., R.D.

Tofu and Kale Quiche

Serves 4 to 6

1/2 teaspoon canola oil
1/2 cup chopped green onions
8 ounces firm tofu, crumbled
1 cup packed finely chopped kale or turnip greens
1 cup grated soy cheese
1/2 cup chopped red bell peppers
1/2 teaspoon salt
1/2 teaspoon turmeric
1 9-inch store-bought pastry pie shell, prepared according to package
   directions

In a small, nonstick skillet, heat oil over medium heat. Add green onions and sauté for 3 minutes. Add remaining ingredients to skillet and mix together until soy cheese begins to soften and kale wilts slightly.

Transfer mixture to prepared pie shell. Bake quiche in preheated oven for 40 minutes.

Recipe from CalciYum! *by David and Rachelle Bronfman*

Desserts

Banana Dream Pie

Serves 8

1 vegan pie crust
1/2 cup sugar or other sweetener
5 tablespoons cornstarch
2 cups soy- or rice milk
1/2 teaspoon salt
1 teaspoon vanilla extract
1/2 pound firm tofu
2 ripe bananas
2 tablespoons coarsely chopped almonds

Prepare the crust according to directions. Cool.

Mix the sugar and cornstarch in a saucepan, then stir in the soy- or rice milk and salt. Cook over medium heat, stirring constantly, until very thick. Remove from the heat and stir in the vanilla. Drain the tofu and blend it in a food processor until it is totally smooth, then add the pudding and blend until smooth.

Slice the bananas into thin rounds over the cooled crust. Spread the tofu mixture on top.

Toast the chopped almonds in a 375°F oven until lightly browned, about 10 minutes, then sprinkle evenly over the pie. Refrigerate until completely chilled, at least 2 hours.

Recipe from Eat Right, Live Longer *by Neal D. Barnard, M.D.;*
recipe by Jennifer Raymond

Banana Pudding

Serves 4; makes 3 cups

10 ounces soft tofu
6 ounces firm tofu
2 small very ripe bananas
1/2 cup granulated sugar
1/4 cup calcium-fortified soymilk, rice milk, almond milk, or oat milk
(continued on next page)

(Banana Pudding continued)
2 teaspoons vanilla

In a blender or food processor, blend all ingredients until creamy and smooth. Pour into small dessert cups and refrigerate for 2 hours. Serve cold.

Recipe adapted from CalciYum! *by David and Rachelle Bronfman.*

Berry Applesauce
Makes 2 cups

Serve this applesauce hot or cold.

2 cups peeled, cored, and chopped apples
2 cups strawberries, blueberries, or raspberries, fresh or frozen (unsweetened)
1/2 cup frozen concentrate or 3/4 cup fruit juice, such as apple, grape, or pomegranate
cinnamon

In a medium-sized saucepan combine all ingredients. Bring to a simmer, then cover and cook over very low heat for about 25 minutes, or until apples are tender when pierced with a fork. Mash lightly or purée in a food processor, if desired. Sprinkle with cinnamon to serve.

Recipe adapted from Foods That Fight Pain *by Neal Barnard, M.D.;*
recipe by Jennifer Raymond

Chocolate Mousse or Chocolate Mousse Pie
Serves 8

1 cup semi-sweet, non-dairy chocolate chips
1/2 cup soy- or other non-dairy milk
1 package Mori-Nu brand silken tofu (firm or extra firm)
1/3 cup sweetener of your choice
1/2 teaspoon vanilla extract

Combine the chocolate and non-dairy milk in a microwave-safe bowl or double boiler and melt, using gentle heat and stirring often. Remove from heat.

Crumble tofu in a blender or food processor. Add melted chocolate and non-dairy milk, sweetener, and vanilla extract. Process until completely smooth, pausing the blender or food processor to scrape down the sides and under the blade as necessary.

Chill the mixture in serving bowls—or, if desired, a low-fat graham cracker or cookie crust—for at least 1 hour before serving. Garnish with fruit.

Variation: Add a chopped banana to the food processor when you process the tofu and chocolate together.

Fig Spice Cake

Makes 9 squares

This is a moist, flavorful cake to enjoy without guilt.

1 cup cut-up, destemmed figs
1 cup hot water
1/4 cup sunflower oil
1/3 cup molasses
1/3 cup brown sugar, packed
1 cup whole wheat flour
1 cup unbleached flour
2 teaspoons baking powder
1/2 teaspoon baking soda
1 teaspoon cinnamon
1/2 teaspoon nutmeg
1/4 teaspoon ground allspice

Soak figs in water for 1 hour. Drain, reserving 1/3 cup of the soaking liquid. Preheat oven to 350°F, and spray a 9×9-inch pan with cooking spray.

Measure the sunflower oil, molases, brown sugar, and reserved fig soaking liquid into a bowl. Mix, then add the flours, baking powder, baking soda, and spices.

Stir, adding the figs. Pour into the prepared pan and bake 45–50 minutes, until cake begins to pull away from the sides of the pan.

Cool. Cut into nine squares. Dust with a sprinkle of confectioner's sugar if desired.

Recipe from Holiday Diet Cookbook *by Dorothy R. Bates*

Gingered Melon Wedges

Serves 6

1 large cantaloupe
1 scant tablespoon powdered sugar
1/2 teaspoon ground ginger
1 tablespoon candied ginger *(optional)*

Cut melon in half and seed. Then cut each half into chunks.
Stir together the sugar and ground ginger. Add candied ginger if you like.
Sprinkle over melon chunks and chill.

Recipe from The Vegetarian No-Cholesterol Barbecue Cookbook
by Kate Schumann and Virginia Messina, M.P.H., R.D.

Prune Pudding

Serves 3 to 4

1 cup prunes
1 cup water
1/3 cup soymilk or rice milk
3 tablespoons carob powder
2 tablespoons maple syrup

Place prunes and water in a covered saucepan and simmer until tender, about 20 minutes. Allow to cool slightly, then transfer the prunes and any remaining liquid to a blender. Add remaining ingredients and blend until completely smooth. Spoon into small serving dishes and chill for at least 1 hour.

Recipe from Food for Life *by Neal D. Barnard, M.D.;*
recipes by Jennifer Raymond

Pumpkin Custard Pie

Serves 6 to 8

1 1/2 cups soymilk
4 tablespoons cornstarch
1 1/2 cups cooked pumpkin
1/2 cup raw sugar or other sweetener
1/2 teaspoon salt
1 teaspoon ground cinnamon
1/2 teaspoon ground ginger
1/8 teaspoon ground cloves
1 9-inch unbaked pie shell

Preheat the oven to 375°F.

In a large bowl, whisk together the soymilk and cornstarch until smooth, then blend in pumpkin, sweetener, salt, and spices. Pour into pie shell and bake for 45 minutes, or until firm. Cool before cutting.

Recipe from Food for Life *by Neal D. Barnard, M.D.;*
recipe by Jennifer Raymond

Schoolyard Oatmeal Cookies

Makes one dozen cookies

The best darn cookies this side of the playground!

1/2 cup whole wheat pastry flour
1/2 cup quick-cooking rolled oats (not instant)
1/4 teaspoon non-aluminum baking powder (such as Rumford)
1/4 teaspoon ground cinnamon
1/4 cup light molasses or sorghum syrup

(continued on next page)

(Schoolyard Oatmeal Cookies continued)
2 tablespoons canola oil
1 tablespoon water
3/4 teaspoon vanilla extract
1/4 cup walnuts, coarsely chopped
1/4 cup raisins

Preheat the oven to 350° F. Coat a baking sheet with nonstick cooking spray, and set it aside.

Place the flour, rolled oats baking powder, cinnamon, and salt in a small mixing bowl. Stir them together and set aside.

Measure out the molasses or sorghum syrup in a small measuring cup. Then stir in the canola oil, water, and vanilla extract. Mix well. Pour this mixture into the dry ingredients along with the walnuts and raisins. Mix thoroughly.

Drop the dough by 12 rounded spoonfuls onto the prepared baking sheet. Flatten each cookie lightly with the back of a spoon.

Bake the cookies for 12 to 14 minutes or until they are lightly browned.

Transfer the cookies to a cooling rack using a metal spatula. Cool the cookies completely before storing them.

Recipe from Table for Two: Meat- and Dairy-Free Recipes
by Joanne Stepaniak

Summer Fruit Compote
Makes 2 cups

2 cups peeled and sliced fresh peaches (peeling is optional)
2 cups hulled fresh strawberries
1/2 cup white grape juice concentrate or apple juice concentrate

In a large saucepan, combine all ingredients. Bring to a simmer and cook for about 5 minutes, or until fruit just becomes soft. Serve warm or cold by itself or over fruit sorbet or vanilla soy ice cream.

Recipe from Foods That Fight Pain *by Neal D. Barnard, M.D.;*
recipe by Jennifer Raymond

Sweet Potato Pie
Serves 8

3 large sweet potatoes
3 tablespoons oil or non-dairy (vegan) margarine
1/2 cup hot soymilk
egg replacer equivalent to 2 eggs
1/2 cup fructose
(continued on next page)

(Sweet Potato Pie continued)
1/2 teaspoon sea salt
1/2 teaspoon vanilla
1/4 teaspoon nutmeg
1 unbaked vegan pie crust

Steam the sweet potatoes until tender, then peel and mash.

Preheat the oven to 350°F. Place the oil in the hot soymilk, and add to the sweet potatoes. Beat until soft and creamy.

Add the beaten egg replacer, fructose, sea salt, vanilla, and nutmeg to the sweet potato mixture, and mix well. Pour the filling into the crust, and bake for 30 minutes.

Recipe from Vegetarian Cooking for People with Allergies
by Raphael Rettner, D.C.

Sweet Potato Pudding

Makes about 1 1/2 cups

Sweet Potato Pudding is a great way to load up on cancer-fighting beta-carotene for breakfast. It takes just minutes to make if you keep cooked sweet potatoes or yams on hand.

1/3 cup rolled oats
1/2 cup fortified soymilk or rice milk
1 cup cooked sweet potato or yam
1 tablespoon maple syrup
1/4 teaspoon cinnamon

Combine all ingredients in a blender and blend until smooth.

Recipe from Healthy Eating for Life to Prevent and Treat Cancer
by Vesanto Melina, M.S., R.D.

Yam Spiced Muffins

Makes 10 to 12 muffins

2 cups whole-wheat flour or whole wheat pastry flour
1/2 cup sugar
1 tablespoon baking powder
1/2 teaspoon baking soda
1/2 teaspoon salt
1/2 teaspoon cinnamon
1/4 teaspoon nutmeg
1 1/2 cups cooked, mashed yams
1/2 cup water
(continued on next page)

(Yam Spiced Muffins continued)

1/2 cup raisins

Preheat the oven to 375°F.

In a large bowl mix whole wheat flour, sugar, baking powder, baking soda, salt, cinnamon, and nutmeg. Add yams, the water, and raisins; stir until just mixed.

Lightly coat a muffin pan with vegetable oil spray. Fill cups to the top with batter.

Bake for 25 to 30 minutes, or until the top of a muffin bounces back when pressed lightly. Let stand for 1 to 2 minutes before removing from the pan. When cool, store in an airtight container.

Recipe from Foods That Fight Pain *by Neal D. Barnard, M.D.;*
recipe by Jennifer Raymond

Yams with Cranberries and Apples

Serves 8

A beautiful blend of sweet and tart flavors, this recipe is a perfect addition to any meal—for the holidays or otherwise.

4 yams, peeled
1 large green apple, peeled and diced
1 cup raw cranberries
1/2 cup raisins
2 tablespoons raw sugar or other sweetener
1/2 cup orange juice

Preheat oven to 350°F.

Cut peeled yams into 1-inch chunks and place in a large baking dish. Top with diced apple, cranberries, and raisins. Sprinkle with sugar or other sweetener, then pour orange juice over all. Cover and bake for 1 hour and 15 minutes or until yams are tender when pierced with a fork.

Recipe from Food for Life *by Neal D. Barnard, M.D.;*
recipe by Jennifer Raymond

Breakfasts

Baked Oatmeal

Serves 2

1 teaspoon oil
1 1/2 cups oatmeal
2 tablespoons low-fat soymilk powder
1 banana, mashed
1 1/2 cups hot water

Preheat oven to 350°F. Oil a small casserole dish with the oil. Mix the remaining ingredients together in the casserole in the order listed. Bake for 20 minutes.

Recipe from Vegetarian Cooking for People with Allergies
by Raphael Rettner, D.C.

Black Beans with Salsa on Toast

Serves 2

At Maya Caribe in Cancun, Mexico, you can fall out of your hotel bed onto the beach and be served a local breakfast of beans with toast. The salsa is a real eye-opener.

1 cup dry black beans
salt, garlic powder, and cumin to taste
1 teaspoon thinly sliced jalapeños
1 large tomato, diced
1/4 cup diced onions
4 slices of your favorite toast or tortillas

Start with black beans. You can boil them from scratch for about 2 hours after soaking them overnight. Do not undercook. After cooking, season them with salt, garlic powder, and cumin. Or you can make life easier and simply use canned beans (1 15-ounce can).

Heat and mash the beans.

For the salsa, mix the jalapeños, tomatoes, and onions, adjusting amounts to taste.

Serve the beans and salsa on toast or with tortillas.

Recipe from Maya Caribe, Cancun, Mexico, printed in
The Best in the World, *edited by Neal Barnard, M.D.*

Breakfast Rice Pudding

Serves 6

2 cups cooked brown rice
1 1/2 cups vanilla rice milk
3 tablespoons raisins
2 tablespoons maple syrup
1 teaspoon vanilla extract
1/4 teaspoon cinnamon

In a medium-sized saucepan, combine all ingredients and bring to a slow simmer. Cook uncovered, stirring occasionally, for about 20 minutes, or until thick. Serve hot or cold.

Recipe from Foods That Fight Pain *by Neal Barnard, M.D.;
recipe by Jennifer Raymond*

Breakfast Scramble

Serves 4

1/2 teaspoon turmeric
1/4 teaspoon pepper
1/4 teaspoon salt
1 teaspoon parsley flakes, lightly crumbled
2 teaspoons vegetable oil
1/2 medium onion
2 cloves garlic
1/2 green bell pepper, chopped
1/2 red bell pepper, chopped
1 pound tofu, drained

Combine herbs and spices in a small dish. Sauté onion and garlic in oil until tender. Add green and red pepper pieces, and cook until peppers are softened. Crumble the tofu into skillet, sprinkle mixture with combined seasonings, and cook, stirring over medium heat until heated through.

Fruited Breakfast Quinoa

Makes about 3 cups

Quinoa is a highly nutritious grain that was a staple in the diet of the ancient Incas. It has a delicious flavor and a light, fluffy texture. It is important to rinse the grain thoroughly prior to cooking.

1/2 cup uncooked quinoa
1 1/2 cups vanilla rice milk
2 tablespoons raisins
1 cup chopped fresh or canned apricots
1/4 teaspoon vanilla extract
(continued on next page)

(Fruited Breakfast Quinoa continued)

To thoroughly rinse quinoa, cover it with water in a mixing bowl, then rub it between the palms of your hands. Pour off the cloudy liquid through a strainer and then repeat the process two or three more times, until the rinse liquid remains clear.

In a medium-sized saucepan, combine the rinsed and drained quinoa with rice milk. Bring to a slow simmer, then cover and cook for about 15 minutes until the quinoa is tender. Stir in the remaining ingredients, then transfer about 1 1/2 cups to a blender; purée.

Return puréed mixture to the pan and stir to mix. Serve warm or chilled.

Recipe from Foods That Fight Pain *by Neal Barnard, M.D.;*
recipe by Jennifer Raymond

Quick Coffee Cake

Serves 6

1 cup unsifted all-purpose flour
1 cup unsifted whole wheat flour
3/4 cup old-fashioned rolled oats, divided
1/3 cup firmly packed light brown sugar
1 tablespoon baking powder
2 teaspoons ground cinnamon
1/2 teaspoon ground nutmeg
1/4 teaspoon ground ginger
pinch of salt
1/2 cup non-dairy (vegan) margarine, divided
1 cup unsweetened apple juice

Preheat the oven to 350°F. Grease and flour a 9-inch square baking pan.

In a large bowl, combine the flours, 1/2 cup of the oats, sugar, baking powder, cinnamon, nutmeg, ginger, and salt. Remove 1/2 cup of the mixture to a cup or small bowl, and add the remaining 1/4 cup oats. Cut in 2 tablespoons of the margarine; set the mixture aside.

Cut the remaining margarine into the flour mixture in the large bowl. Stir in the apple juice until well combined. Pour the batter into the prepared pan. Top with the reserved oat mixture.

Bake the cake about 40 minutes, or until a knife inserted in center come out clean. Cool to room temperature before serving.

Recipe from The Vegetarian Way *by Virginia Messina, M.P.H., R.D.,*
and Mark Messina, Ph.D.

Spiced Pumpkin Pancakes

Serves 4 to 6

These unusual spiced pancakes are perfect for a weekend brunch. Top with thinly sliced fresh fruit, such as peaches, strawberries, or bananas, and hot maple syrup.

1/2 cup canned puréed pumpkin
1/2 cup yellow cornmeal
1/2 cup unbleached flour
1/4 cup brown sugar
1 teaspoon baking powder
1/4 teaspoon salt
1/2 teaspoon pumpkin pie spice
1 teaspoon grated orange peel
2 teaspoons finely chopped candied ginger *(optional)*
1/4 cup water
1 tablespoon vegetable oil
3/4 cup plain or vanilla soymilk

Combine the pumpkin with the dry ingredients. Mix water, oil, and soy-milk and add to pumpkin mixture. Beat just until smooth. Heat griddle or frying pan and oil lightly. Use about 1/4 cup of batter for each pancake; cook until bubbles appear, then turn. Remove when pancakes are golden and slightly firm to the touch.

Recipe from The Vegetarian No-Cholesterol Family-Style Cookbook *by Kate Schumann and Virginia Messina, M.P.H., R.D.*

Tofu French Toast

Makes 6 pieces of toast

8 ounces low-fat tofu
1/2 cup water
1 teaspoon sweetener (molasses or maple syrup)
1/2 teaspoon cinnamon
1 banana
6 slices whole wheat bread

Mix all ingredients except the bread in a blender until smooth. Pour blended mixture into a shallow dish. Dip the whole wheat bread into mixture and cook on a nonstick pan.

Beverages

Breakfast Shakes

Each recipe makes about 2 cups

Creamy Berry Smoothie:
1 banana
1/2 cup frozen berries
1 cup calcium-fortified vanilla soymilk (or other milk alternative)
2 tablespoons maple syrup *(optional)*
2 tablespoons calcium-fortified orange juice from frozen concentrate

Not-So-Creamy Berry Smoothie:
2 cups frozen berries
2 tablespoon maple syrup *(optional)*
2 tablespoon calcium-fortified orange juice from frozen concentrate
water as needed

Green Goodie:
1 cup pineapple juice
1 cup calcium-fortified vanilla soymilk (or other milk alternative)
10 frozen peach slices
1 banana
1/4 cup cherries, pitted, or raspberries
2 teaspoons maple syrup *(optional)*
1 heaping teaspoon spirulina
ice, as needed, to chill and thicken

Place all ingredients in a blender. Blend at high speed until smooth. (You'll have to stop the blender occasionally and move the unblended fruit to the center with a spatula to get your smoothie smooth.)

Cranberry Papaya Juice

Makes 2 cups

1 cup orange juice (preferably calcium fortified)
1/2 of a ripe papaya, seeded, peeled, and chopped
1/2 cup cranberry juice
1 1/2 teaspoons lemon juice

In a blender, process all ingredients until smooth. Refrigerate and serve cold.

Recipe from CalciYum! by David and Rachelle Bronfman

Easy Almond Nut Milk

1/2 cup almonds
1 1/2 cups boiling water

Blend almonds and boiling water together for about 3 minutes at a high speed. Strain through muslin or cheesecloth. The remaining pulp can be used in vegetable/nut loaves or burgers. Shake milk well before serving.

Recipe from Meatless Meals for Working People
by Debra Wasserman and Charles Stahler

Fresh Collard-Apple Juice

Makes 1 cup

2 sweet apples, cored and quartered
1 1/4 cups packed collard greens (leaves and steams), rinsed

Add a few slices of apple to juicer then some of the collard greens. Extract juice. Repeat this process until ingredients are used up. (Finish off with apple slices to make juice flow smoothly through the juicer.) Discard solids.

Recipe from CalciYum! *by David and Rachelle Bronfman*

Sauces and Gravies

Chunky Ratatouille Sauce

Serves 6

1 large eggplant, cut into 1-inch chunks
2 stalks celery, chopped
2 small onions, chopped
8 ounces of cremini mushrooms
6 cloves garlic, minced
1/2 cup red wine
1/4–1/2 cup water
1 teaspoon Italian seasoning
1/2 teaspoon thyme
1/2 teaspoon black pepper (add more to taste)
1 15-ounce can fire-roasted tomatoes

Soak eggplant chunks in salted water for 10 minutes. Drain, rinse, and drain again. Braise onion, celery, and garlic in 1/4 cup of red wine. When the vegetables are soft, add the eggplant chunks and 1/4 cup of water. Simmer, stirring occasionally, until the eggplant is soft (about 8 to 10 minutes). Add more water if necessary to keep mixture from drying out. Add mushrooms, herbs and spices, remaining wine, and tomatoes. Simmer for 5 minutes. Serve over pasta shells, brown rice, or your favorite grain.

Recipe from PCRM Weight Loss Study Cooking Demonstration; contributed by PCRM nutrition director Amy Lanou, Ph.D.

Chunky Red Lentil Tomato Sauce

Serves 8

1 onion, diced
2 to 3 cloves garlic, minced
1 large carrot, sliced diagonally
1 stalk broccoli, chopped
1 cup mushrooms (fresh or canned), sliced
1/2 cup sweet green pepper, diced
1 small zucchini, sliced or grated
1 28-ounce can stewed tomatoes, whole or diced
1 28-ounce can prepared tomato sauce

(continued on next page)

(Chunky Red Lentil Tomato Sauce continued)

1 cup water
1/2 to 1 cup dried red lentils
2 tablespoons fresh basil leaves or 2 teaspoons dried basil leaves
2 tablespoons fresh oregano leaves or 2 teaspoons dried oregano leaves

Place all the ingredients in a saucepan or slow cooker, and stir.

If using the stove-top method, bring the ingredients to a boil, turn the heat down, and simmer the sauce for about 1 hour or more. If using a slow cooker, cook on low for 6 to 8 hours or on high for about 4 hours. Serve with your favorite pasta or spaghetti squash.

From Becoming Vegetarian *by Vesanto Melinda,*
Brenda Davis, and Victoria Harrison

Garlicky Tahini Gravy

Serves 3 to 4

2 cloves garlic, minced
1 teaspoon canola or olive oil
1/2 cup tahini (sesame butter)
1/4 cup tamari or soy sauce

In a small saucepan, sauté garlic in oil. Whisk in tahini and tamari, and whisk until blended and creamy. Serve hot.

Recipe by Jennifer Brewer

Mushrooms with Barbecue Sauce

Serves 4

1 small yellow onion, finely chopped
1/4 cup water
12 ounces button or cremini mushrooms, sliced
1/2 cup barbecue sauce

Braise onions in 1/4 cup water for 3–4 minutes. Add mushrooms and continue cooking for 4–5 more minutes. Add barbecue sauce and cook until sauce is desired thickness. Serve over veggie burgers, potatoes, or any whole grain.

Recipe from PCRM's Nutrition and Cooking Classes for Cancer Survivors;
contributed by PCRM nutrition director Amy Lanou, Ph.D.

Mushroom Gravy

Serves 4 to 8

12 ounces button or cremini mushrooms
2 teaspoons olive oil
1–2 tablespoons soy sauce *(optional)*
3 tablespoons flour
1–2 cups vegetable stock, divided
1 teaspoon Italian seasoning salt and black pepper, to taste

Clean and slice mushrooms, then sauté in oil until soft (about 5 minutes). Mix flour with 1/4 cup of stock or water until smooth (whisk together in a bowl or shake it in a small plastic container with a tight fitting lid). Add remaining stock to the mushrooms along with the soy sauce and about 1/2 the flour mixture. Bring gravy to a simmer for 3 to 5 minutes, stirring regularly. If the gravy is not thick enough for your taste, add the remaining flour mixture and continue heating and stirring until it thickens. Serve immediately.

Additional Resources

Nutrition Information

Barnard, Neal. *Food for Life*. Harmony Books, 1993.

Barnard, Neal. *Eat Right, Live Longer*. Harmony Books, 1995.

Barnard, Neal. *Foods That Fight Pain*. Harmony Books, 1998.

Barnard, Neal. *Turn off the Fat Genes*. Harmony Books, 2001.

Davis, Brenda, and Melina, Vesanto. *Becoming Vegan*. Book Publishing Co., 2000.

McDougall, John. *The McDougall Program*. Plume Books, 1991.

Moran, Victoria. *The Love-Powered Diet*. New World Library, 1992.

Ornish, Dean. *Dr. Dean Ornish's Program for Reversing Heart Disease*. Random House, 1990.

Ornish, Dean. *Eat More, Weigh Less*. HarperCollins, 1993.

Physicians Committee for Responsible Medicine with Melina, Vesanto. *Healty Eating for Life to Prevent and Treat Cancer*, John Wiley & Sons, 2002.

Stepaniak, Joanne. *The Vegan Sourcebook*. McGraw-Hill, 2000.

World Cancer Research Fund and American Institute for Cancer Research. *Food, Nutrition, and the Prevention of Cancer: A Global Perspective*. Washington, D.C.: American Institute for Cancer Research, 1997.

Cookbooks

Barnard, Neal, ed. *The Best in the World*. Physicians Committee for Responsible Medicine, 1998.

Barnard, Tanya, and Kramer, Sarah. *How it all Vegan*. Arsenal Pulp Press, Ltd., 1999.

Bennett, Jannequin. *Very Vegetarian*. Rutledge Hill Press, 2001.

Bronfman, David and Rachelle. *CalciYum!* Bromedia, 1998.

Davis, Brenda; Grogan, Bryanna Clark; and Stepaniak, Joanne. *Dairy-Free and Delicious*. Book Publishing Company, 2001.

Keller, Jennifer, ed. *The Best in the World II*. Physicians Committee for Responsible Medicine, 2002.

Kornfeld, Myra. *The Voluptuous Vegan*. Clarkson N. Potter, 2000.

McDougall, Mary and John. *The McDougall Quick & Easy Cookbook*. Plume, 1999.

Oser, Marie. *The Enlightened Kitchen*. John Wiley & Sons, 2002.

Raymond, Jennifer. *Fat-Free & Easy*. Heart & Soul Publications, 1997.
Sass, Lorna. *Lorna Sass' Complete Vegetarian Kitchen*. HarperCollins, 1995.
Stepaniak, Joanne. *Table for Two*. Book Publishing Company, 1996.
Stepaniak, Joanne. *The Uncheese Cookbook*. Book Publishing Co., 1994.
Stepaniak, Joanne. *Vegan Deli*. Book Publishing Company, 2001.

Videotapes

Barnard, Neal. *Foods for Cancer Prevention and Survival* (videotape, 45 minutes). Physicians Committee for Responsible Medicine.
Eating Right for Cancer Survival (videotape of eight nutrition lectures, 1 hour 43 minutes). The Cancer Project.

E-Newsletter

Breaking Medical News is a free service of the Physicians Committee for Responsible Medicine, bringing you news from the latest research studies, often before they are available through Medline or other computerized retrieval systems. To subscribe, visit *www.pcrm.org*.

The Survivor's Handbook: Eating Right for Cancer Survival,
a production of The Cancer Project, is made possible by:

A Sparrow's Song Foundation

The Lance Armstrong Foundation

Mental Insight Foundation

PacifiCare Foundation

Help us win the battle against cancer

About The Cancer Project

With over one million people being diagnosed with cancer in the United States each year—and many more cases in other countries across the globe—there is an urgent need for a new direction in battling this disease. The Cancer Project is a collaborative effort of physicians, researchers, and nutritionists who have joined together to educate the public on how a healthy diet can protect us from cancer and help us regain our health once cancer has been diagnosed.

The Key Is Information

Most Americans do not yet have the facts about the relationship between nutrition and cancer. Surveys conducted by Opinion Research Corporation International have repeatedly found that most people have never heard of links between diet and cancer. In other words, information has not been getting to people who need it.

That is why we established The Cancer Project—to disseminate life-saving information as widely as possible and keep it from being buried in medical libraries.

Getting the Word Out

The Cancer Project distributes information on reducing cancer risk and, when cancer has been diagnosed, how diet and other factors may help improve survival. Vital information has reached millions of individuals and families through brochures, television advertisements, Web-based information, and nutrition and cooking classes.

The Cancer Project also distributes thousands of pieces of information to health professionals at conferences and conventions. We stress the need for more effective educational efforts on nutrition and cancer prevention. Televised public service announcements are released nationally twice a year. The Cancer Project's Food for Life nutrition and cooking class series for cancer prevention and survival is being taught all over the country to help individuals understand how and why to cook nutritiously. The classes not only help individuals understand how and why to cook nutritously, they also act as a lighthearted support group for cancer survivors or those who have been touched by cancer in some way. *The Survivor's Handbook* and the companion video, *Eating Right for Cancer Survival,* were developed to accompany the class series, but they can also be used on their own to help cancer survivors or individuals interested in cancer prevention have access to this vital information at home.

Your Help Makes It Possible!

The success of our efforts depends entirely on the resources available for producing and distributing printed information, funding our research, working with the media, staffing booths at medical conferences, and teaching our Food for Life nutrition and cooking classes. Both large and small contributions make an enormous difference.

If you wish to support our work to advance cancer prevention and survival through nutrition education and research, you may donate online at *www.CancerProject.org*. If you prefer, you can mail or phone in your contribution to:

THE CANCER PROJECT
5100 Wisconsin Ave. NW, Suite 400
Washington, DC 20016
Phone: 202-244-5038